BACK PAIN RELIEF:
THE ULTIMATE GUIDE

BACK PAIN RELIEF: THE ULTIMATE GUIDE

A COMPREHENSIVE BACK PAIN MANAGEMENT PROGRAM

ROBERT H. MILLER and CHRISTINE A. OPIE

Foreword by
DR. WILLIAM BROSE
Founder and Former Director
Stanford University Pain Management Center

CAPRA PRESS
SANTA BARBARA

Cover design and book design: Frank Goad
Cover photograph: Wayne Yentis

Library of Congress Cataloging-in-Publication Data

Miller , Robert H. , 1941 Feb. 16
  Back pain relief : a comprehensive back pain management program /
by Robert H. Miller and Christine A. Opie ; with a foreword by William Brose.
      p.   cm.
  "A unique pain management program drawn from one patient's
successful treatment at Stanford University Medical Center Pain
Management Service and complementary medicine pain relief methods
featuring easy-to-follow instructions to assist in mastering the physical
and mental means of pain relief."
  Includes index.
  ISBN 0-88496-418-3 (pbk . : alk . paper)
  1. Backache—Popular works. 2. Backache—Treatment. 3. Backache—
Alternative treatment.   I. Opie , Christine A., 1953-
II. Title
RD771.B217M55   1997
617.5'64—dc21   96-47953
                                                                      CIP

CAPRA ❦ PRESS
P.O. Box 2068
Santa Barbara, CA 93120

DEDICATION

ROBERT H. MILLER
dedicates this book to the following members of the health care
community who have played a material role in his recovery,
as well as to the members of his family,
wife Bonnie and son Jason:
Dr. William Brose
Dr. William Longton
Dr. David Gutlove
Dr. James Massey
Dr. Howard Hoffman
Dr. Melvin Friedman
Dr. Steven Raffin
Dr. Peter Grossman
Dr. Malcom Kushner
Susan Tingely, physical therapist
Steven Anderson, physical therapist
Andrew Wright, Feldenkrais practitioner
Jane Pitzinger, physical therapist
Julie Rogers, Somatics Educator

CHRISTINE A. OPIE
dedicates this book to:
Monica Leone, "down under" who started me on the path to this book,
to Ed, my brother, who let me fill up his hard drive with countless
versions of the manuscript, and to LLP who guides me always
and without whom this book would not be.

Finally both authors would like to acknowledge and thank David Dahl
of Capra Press for his skillful editing

DISCLAIMER

The authors and publisher of this book are not rendering medical advice, attempting to diagnose any medical condition, or prescribing any techniques as treatment in this book. The advice and procedures described and offered for the reader's use are intended to augment and enhance professional medical treatment, not replace it. It is essential that you discuss and obtain approval for all aspects of these programs with your physician, as well as with other health care professionals treating your condition, before undertaking any part of the programs. If you choose to use any techniques or exercises presented in this book without first talking with and obtaining approval from your physician, you do so at your own risk. The authors and publisher disclaim any legal, financial, or moral responsibility for any adverse effects resulting from any of the information contained in the book or CDs.

ABOUT THE AUDIO CDs

The two audio compact discs referred to in the text are available for purchase from the authors. Please see Appendix E for their contents and ordering information, as well as the order form at the end of the book. While the pain relief programs described herein can be accomplished without the aid of the CDs, the authors highly recommend their purchase and use. The CDs will greatly accelerate the learning process involved in using the pain relief techniques and will enhance their effectiveness. Original music has been composed by Pat Parr, and the voice on the discs is co-author Christine Opie.

CONTENTS

FOREWORD

WILLIAM G. BROSE, M.D.
Associate Professor of Anesthesia
Founder and Former Director, Stanford University Medical Center
Pain Management Service

PAIN IS ENDEMIC IN OUR SOCIETY. Each year millions of Americans are afflicted with chronic pain, including low back pain, headaches, arthritis, and many more uncommon but no less painful medical conditions. The early identification of pain as a symptom by the medical community has led to gross undertreatment of most chronic pain conditions by physicians in modern medical practice. After all, as physicians we don't treat symptoms; we are taught to treat diseases. The biomedical model that educates physicians and, in fact, has permeated much of the fabric of American society, fosters the undertreatment of pain we currently experience today. As a part of Western scientific method, when one identifies a problem, the first goal in resolving the problem is to identify its cause. Identifying causes for medical problems has led to some tremendous values in health care, including the identification of infectious bacteria, viruses and other organisms which cause disease. The subsequent development of specific antibiotic and vaccine treatments to virtually eradicate such parasitic and infectious diseases is due to that biomedical research. However, while we have had success in some ventures using this search for the cause, in other areas medicine has far too little information and far too little knowledge to impact such a positive outcome. Witness the problems of diabetes, arthritis, cancer, heart disease, all of which afflict millions of patients in the United States every day. In some of these conditions, we understand the underlying pathogenesis and etiology and yet are unable to provide a cure. In others, we as yet do not possess the knowledge to even clearly delineate pathophysiology, let alone the inciting cause.

The failure to be able to "cure" chronic pain is recognized by most physicians and accepted by many patients. However, the problem in chronic pain is all too similar to any other chronic medical condition. Since we do not know how to cure it, what can we do? Physicians are taught to view chronic pain as an extension of the acute pain warning system. As such, the pain tells us that something may pose a threat to our lives or the integrity of our bodies. Chronic pain, however, provides no such threat and this awareness should help physicians as well as patients to recognize that chronic pain is a separate disease, which, like other chronic diseases, needs to be appropriately managed. Unlike the quest for the elusive cure of chronic pain, which continues to evade us, by viewing pain as a chronic disease, one can look for successful strategies to help reduce the impact of this disease on a patient's life.

In the Pain Management Center at Stanford the view of pain as a chronic disease is well supported. For this reason, the orientation of patient care within the Pain Service is that of an outcome-oriented approach helping to individualize the treatments of each patient to achieve the specific outcomes they desire. By assessing the multitude of impacts that chronic pain has had on patients' lives, interrupting their vocational, social, and recreational pursuits, increasing their reliance on health care resources, as well as contributing to their overall physical and mental health, physician providers can assess areas of greatest need for patients and by working with them, identify the most successful management strategies to reverse the impacts of pain on their lives.

Bob Miller was one such patient who identified himself to me in his first visit in February 1994. Miller had been afflicted with low back pain, intermittently for nearly a year. While initially he had seen a number of specialists, each seeking the "holy grail" of a cure for his pain, time and time again these providers failed to identify the sole causative agent. Their failures were not the failures of individual doctors in treating a single patient, but rather should be recognized as the failures of a symptom-oriented biomedical model failing to provide adequate diagnostic and treatment tools for conditions as complex as Miller's low back pain. Unfortunately, in the multiple failures that he had experienced with the medical community, the message that was being reinforced was not that his back pain was real, but perhaps too complicated or too multifactorial for the current state of medical knowledge to clearly identify a solid cause. Instead, he was left with the impression that either there must be something sinister accounting for his low back pain that had yet to be identified by any of these skilled practitioners, or that his pain, in fact, was fictitious and presenting itself as a primary manifestation of some underlying mental disorder.

After first going through a series of appropriate steps in medical and psychological evaluation, the providers in the Pain Service attempted to educate Miller that his back pain was not evidence of some sinister, underlying pathology that represented a threat to his life, nor was it evidence of some smoldering mental disorder that would eventually lead to his being diagnosed as "crazy." Instead, we educated him to the multifactorial nature of his low back pain, which included elements of muscular spasm, disk and facet inflammation, as well as super-imposed psychological stressors, all of which combined to make this a chronic pain condition. By identifying the impacts that this chronic painful condition had had on his life, and working with him to specify the areas where he would like to see the most immediate change, we initiated treatments that engaged him, from medical, rehabilitative and psychological perspectives. By having Miller accept the responsibility for measurement and monitoring of his changes with the various medical and non-medical components of treatment, he was quickly able to identify those elements of care which were linked most directly to improvement of outcome.

Once this process was initiated, Bob Miller began his own quest to identify the specific components of non-medical management that would take him to the highest levels of productivity he had seen in his lifetime. After working some months at half-time due to his chronic back pain problem, he was able to return to his demanding career as an attorney and director of a federal government agency regional office. In addition to the demands of his full-time position, he was functioning so well that after extensive study and research in the areas of pain management and alternative medicine, he co-authored this comprehensive book. Moreover after 315 hours of instruction, he became a California Certified Holistic Health Counselor and in this capacity has assisted others in managing their pain.

The success of Miller's program for managing his low back pain documented in this book should stand as a reassurance to all patients afflicted with chronic painful conditions to help them recognize that if they can engage in the same type of introspective process, they too can learn to manage their chronic back pain. As a secondary benefit of Miller's involvement in the Pain Management Service at Stanford, this book provides a unique and well-structured presentation of the myriad different non-medical management techniques for chronic pain. By picking up and reviewing this text, not only can patients with chronic low back pain identify and learn from someone who has transcended his problem, but moreover they can use specific instructions and self-help tools provided with the book to integrate these same successful management strategies into their own treatment armamentarium.

As a physician I am pleased to see the progress that Bob Miller has been able to make in his personal battle with chronic pain, and moreover I am thankful to him for chronicling and cataloging the treatments he identified for chronic pain, which hopefully will provide similar benefit to back pain sufferers everywhere.

CHAPTER 1

OVERVIEW AND GETTING STARTED

Why This Book Was Written

IN MAY 1993, while lifting a stereo unit out of a car, I fell on my right buttocks. Three hours later, a searing pain traveled down my right leg and, after three days, attacked my lower and mid back and buttocks.

So began a nine-month journey to family doctors, osteopaths, chiropractors, physical therapists, orthopedists, and neurosurgeons. Although each health care professional was competent in his field and prescribed traditional back exercises and moderate doses of anti-inflammatory medicines, I did not get better.

The burning pain traveled continuously up and down my entire back and soon dominated my life. Sometimes my muscles were so tight that my back felt like a board. Every day was the same no matter what I did. Indeed I was unable to work full days. Although x-ray, CAT-scan and MRI studies showed moderately bulging disks, two neurosurgeons concluded that surgery was not indicated. It seemed I was stuck with the pain. My mood soured.

Something had to be done. I hurt all the time and my life was miserable. After further discussion with some medical professionals who had been treating me, they concluded that I should enroll in a pain clinic as a last resort. It was left to me to find the appropriate one. I spoke to each pain clinic in the Northern California Bay Area and felt that for my needs the Stanford Pain Management Service would be the best because it would evaluate my situation and offer a structured, on-going treatment plan.

In early February 1994 my first appointment at Stanford marked a truly eventful day: the beginning of a turn-around in reducing my pain and recommencing my life. I was particularly fortunate because the physician assigned to my case was Dr. William Brose, Founder and Director of the Pain Management Service. During a three-hour consultation, Dr. Brose examined me thoroughly and inquired about my present situation. With Dr. Brose's guidance a four-part program was developed: 1. physical therapy; 2. psychological evaluation and therapy to learn pain management skills; 3. appropriate medication; and 4. finally and most importantly, a goal phase was designed. As the cornerstone of my program, it required me to set and reach recreational, social, exercise, and pain management/control goals on a daily and weekly basis. Within two months, the results were dramatic. I hurt significantly less and resumed full-time work. Most importantly, I was able to live a normal life again.

During this time I developed an avid interest in complementary medicine. I found it enhanced my treatment at Stanford with surprisingly positive results. I was amazed I could control pain through hypnosis or by pressing acupressure points on my hands. The more I read and researched, the more obliged I felt to share the information and techniques that had so dramatically helped me. I knew in the United States alone some 70 million people have suffered back pain for many years. Indeed, my interest was so great that I enrolled in and successfully completed a course to become a California Certified Holistic Health Counselor just prior to the completion of this book.

Simply writing another book about back pain would not do, for a number had already been written. While helpful, many were difficult to follow and were not written in a lucid style, and virtually all were written by professionals in the field. Therefore, I decided a book that would truly help required three concepts:
• *It had to be simple and to the point.*
• *It needed a methodology that would serve as a coach.*
• *It had to be written by a patient successful in the management of back pain.*
Also, to be easily read and understood, a format was developed to establish:
• *What a pain relieving technique is.*
• *Why it works.*
• *How it is done.*

Additionally, other pain relief books provide the reader with exercises and techniques with only the aid of written instructions. In this book, certain critical skills and techniques (such as meditation or self-hypnosis) are presented with an audio "coach" on CD, walking the reader through instructions, ensuring that those skills are learned easily and successfully. *(Please see last page of book for information on obtaining the CDs. As useful as the CDs are, they are not absolutely essential to a successful application of the programs described herein. Also, see note at beginning of book "About The CDs").*

Fortunately, a number of years ago, I met Christine Opie when I took a self-hypnosis class. Christine, a Master Hypnotist and college English instructor, was also interested in alternative healing methods. Christine's soothing voice will guide you through many aspects of this pain relief program on the CDs. Her deep sense of commitment and her teaching experience greatly strengthen the concepts behind this book.

Why was this book written? It was written to share valuable and helpful information with both back pain sufferers and health care professionals who may have been frustrated by the difficulty of treating chronic back pain. We hope the detailed methods and programs in this book will substantially relieve or eliminate chronic back pain, and also make pain sufferers' lives fun and productive again, giving them a renewed enthusiasm for life.

Even before publication, the power of this book to concretely improve back pain sufferers' lives was demonstrated. Author Miller sent draft copies of several chapters to a colleague who had a herniated disk and was suffering significant pain and depression. Some months later, that same colleague wrote to Miller expressing great appreciation and gratitude for the relief he had found using some of the physical and mental techniques from this book. The colleague went on to say that the "holistic approach made a great deal of sense," and that the techniques and information he had been given "enabled [him] to successfully manage [his] pain and finally reach a point where [he is] relatively pain free." Not only was he able to *reduce his pain levels by 95% within a matter of months*, but the affirmations also improved his frame of mind. This testament should provide a great deal of hope and desire to keep reading!

Why This Program Is Unique

Those reading this book as chronic sufferers, or those engaged in the healing arts, may ask what is so different or unique about this book; a key question with many answers:

• It is written from the perspective of a patient who has endured significant pain and personally understands the trauma it can bring to a person's life.

• The book is drawn in part from a program developed by some of the best pain management specialists in the world at the Stanford Pain Management Service.

• Many aspects of the program come from independent research and education in proven centuries-old holistic medicine techniques.

• The book is written in easy-to-understand language that anyone can easily apply.

• Detailed illustrations accompany the text making instructions easy to follow.
• A series of CDs, with verbal instructions and appropriate music, lead you through important pain relief methods. (See Appendix E for instructions on ordering the CDs.) While learning the techniques in this book is possible with only the text for guidance, mastering such healing techniques as hypnosis, deep breathing, meditation, Feldenkrais and Somatics will be far easier with an audio "coach."
• There are three recommended programs: a long form, a short form and a design-your-own one, allowing you to tailor a plan to specific needs. Each is integrated, combining all elements of successful pain management strategies, as well as being easy to follow with daily charts.
• The best reason: The program should *significantly reduce* and in some cases *eliminate* pain.

These then are a few reasons why the programs are unique, but how and why do they work? Pain levels should be reduced because the programs:

• change the attitude towards pain.
• strengthen muscles and make them more flexible
• teach physical and mental means to control and potentially eliminate pain.
• help develop interests and a life program through goal setting/accomplishment.
• offer numerous holistic alternatives to reduce or eliminate pain.
• present the primary causes of pain and ways to deal with the causes
• make you the master of the pain, instead of being its victim.

Important Words of Advice Before You Start

First, we'd like to emphasize that this book does *not* attempt to diagnose or treat back pain. Only a physician can do that. Rather, it is a chronicling of various modalities that one patient used to reduce, relieve, control, and on many occasions eliminate his pain. Through experience, research, and 315 hours of training as a California Certified Holistic Health Counselor, author Miller was able to reduce his pain significantly and return to a full, active life.

We cannot account for each back pain situation. Be sure to discuss with your physician, and obtain approval to use, any pain relief methods presented here. Although pain relief techniques featured in this book have not been approved by the Stanford Pain Management Service, the goal setting concept and much of the exercise program were prescribed by doctors and physical therapists at Stanford. Most of the featured pain relief methods and many of the goal activities were done with the knowledge of doctors at Stanford, who were supportive of complementary medicine techniques as long as they were effective and not otherwise harmful. Indeed, the doctors were supportive of "what worked" in Miller's pain management program.

How To Use The Book

In order to get an overview and initial understanding of the physical and mental means of pain control *before* diving into a program, we suggest first reading the book from cover to cover to understand the theory and goals of the program. Buying this book demonstrates a wish to take a more proactive approach to dealing with chronic pain. How should you approach the program? The answer: slowly and carefully. We are going to recommend certain programs, but they will not incorporate each and every means of physical and mental means of pain control. However, reading the book will provide specific knowledge of many means of pain control to use in addition to the recommended plans. Each of us is different and what works for one might not work for another. If you wish to modify the recommended programs, it will be helpful to know which means of pain control can be substituted for those in a recommended plan.

After reading the entire book, carefully review Chapter 28 on the recommended programs. In reading that chapter, please refer back to the chapters which spell out the aspects of the recommended programs. Once you have decided on elements of the programs you think will be helpful and will feel comfortable using, *discuss them with your physician and obtain his/her approval* to ensure they will not aggravate your condition.

After obtaining your doctor's clearance, practice the recommended techniques, and be sure to master each technique before proceeding to the next. It may take about a week to read the book and practice before actually starting.

An Important Word About Expectations and Progress

These programs take practice, time, and patience. There is no overnight cure. It is important not to expect one. Your chronic back pain condition has probably been going on for many months or years. While you should always think positively and hope for the best, keep things in perspective. We believe there will be a healthy change in attitude and some reduction in pain in the first weeks. Pain control may follow within the next few weeks. It is important not to give up or give way to frustration.

Do not raise expectation levels too high at first and do not have a negative attitude about setbacks. Be assured that the techniques described in the book *work*. They are based upon actual experience and represent the best and latest thinking of professionals in the pain management field.

Pain Management Versus Pain Cure

Many have purchased this book hoping the techniques and means of pain control will totally and instantaneously eliminate back pain. For some that may be the case. For others, while pain may not be eliminated, it may decrease significantly enough to get life back on track. Our minimum goal is to restore back pain sufferers to more functional lives. Pain should be significantly reduced and you will learn how to have a life *you* control as opposed to a life controlled and limited by pain. Don't be discouraged if an immediate and total cure does not occur. Be pleased about learning to manage pain and taking steps in the right direction.

The Role of Your Doctor

Your doctor should play an important role in the program. Why, you ask, especially if a doctor hasn't helped much? While the concepts we suggest are utilized in pain clinics throughout the nation, certain exercises, vitamins and supplements, as well as specific physical or mental techniques for pain control, might not be right for everyone. After designing a personal program, discuss it with your physician to ensure that it is medically sound. In all probability he or she will approve and be pleased to work with you on a proactive approach to managing pain.

Share this book with your physician, so ultimately you both can forge a treatment partnership. Our experience has been that many physicians, other than pain management specialists, are not trained in sophisticated pain management techniques. No doubt your physician will be interested to learn about many of the mental and physical means of pain control discussed in this text.

If your physician has not prescribed pain medicine, a prescription for it should be discussed as part of the overall program. Clinics often prescribe medication to give patients sufficient relief to get started on a pain management program. The efficacy and value of medication should be judged by how well it supports functioning and following a regime, and not necessarily by how much relief the medication provides. In other words, if the medication provides maximum relief, but makes you so groggy that you can do nothing but sleep or lie around, then it is not particularly conducive to learning how to manage pain or returning to full function. However, medication may be required for only a short period. The chosen program to relieve or eliminate pain should show dramatic results within a few weeks. We are confident that your doctor will support efforts to use self-help techniques to manage pain.

Choosing Your Physician or Complementary Health Care Provider
This book emphasizes the importance of working in partnership with health care professionals. A qualified, experienced, knowledgeable, and caring doctor is very important. If you already have such a doctor, wonderful. However, if you need to choose a doctor, the following questions will be useful in selecting a physician or complementary medicine practitioner. (Please note, we are *not* recommending a complementary medicine practitioner *instead* of a physician. However, you may want to choose a complementary health care practitioner to *enhance,* not replace, treatment from a physician.) When selecting a physician, ask yourself:
• Has this doctor treated patients with chronic pain problems? If so, is he/she comfortable in doing so? Has the doctor been successful in treating these patients?
• What is the doctor's specialty? Is it relevant to your pain care needs?
• Has the doctor had any special training or education in treating chronic pain or back pain issues?
• How does the doctor feel about the value of psychotherapy, hypnosis, meditation, and acupuncture or acupressure in dealing with chronic pain? Is he/she open-minded about these practices and would he/she support you in using these methods as an adjunct to your treatment with him/her?
• Does the doctor see you as a whole person not just a hurting back?
• Will this doctor be an advocate for you?
• Has the doctor published papers or spoken at conferences on your type of problem?
• Does the doctor mind if you get a second opinion or if you verify his/her advice?
• Does he/she encourage you to research your problem?
• Does the doctor spend as much time with you as you need or is he/she always rushed?
• Does the office staff treat patients with kindness and respect?

Selecting a Complementary Health Care Practitioner

There is a wide variety of alternative health practitioners, including massage therapists, Chinese herbalists, hypnotherapists, and acupuncturists. These practitioners vary widely in quality and qualifications and in methods and techniques. Screen a potential health practitioner as carefully, if not more carefully than a physician. When choosing a complementary health care practitioner, ask yourself:

• What does the practitioner think about the practice of allopathic medicine? Look for someone who respects modern medical practice and science and wants to be part of a *team* treating you. A practitioner who holds modern medical practice in contempt or has a "us vs. them" attitude is not the best bet.

• What kind of formal training does the person have? Did he/she go to accredited, reputable schools?

• Does the person have the appropriate licenses or certifications in his/her treatment specialty?

• Does the practitioner want you to bring your relevant medical records with you for your first session? He/she should.

• Does the person seem grounded and practical or very abstract and vague?

• Is the treatment room clean, private, and comfortable?

• Do you feel safe with this person? Would you trust him/her with private matters?

• Does the practitioner read medical journals as well as journals and literature relevant to his/her practice?

• Ask the practitioner how his treatment specialty will assist your problem?

• Ask the practitioner for references.

• Does the secretary or receptionist seem professional?

The Importance of a Positive Mental Attitude

Significant time is given in later chapters to the importance of a positive attitude in any pain management program. An optimistic mind set is one of the most important factors in pain control. The success of the techniques in this book largely depends on this positive mind set.

So, before reading any further, begin an attitude shift. Strong motivation to succeed is absolutely critical. Remember, thinking positively, and continually imagining that these programs will substantially relieve or eliminate back pain, will make pain relief a reality. The mind is the most important piece of "equipment" for this program.

Devictimizing Your Pain

A school of thought asserts that we create disease and pain in our bodies through negative emotions and thoughts. We may find this hard to accept because it lays responsibility squarely in our laps. Many of us prefer to think that illness and pain happen *to* us.

In this culture, we often put the blame and responsibility for our negative circumstances *outside* of ourselves. Compared to other cultures, ours is a litigious, blame-seeking culture always looking for someone else to be at fault. There has to be a bad guy and a victim, and we carry this image into our views about health and illness. If we are sick or in pain, it's not our fault. We blame bad genes, germs, pesticides, cholesterol, cigarettes, stress, or the guy who forgot to put up a "wet floor" sign, which resulted in a spine-jarring fall.

Now many are probably thinking, "What do you mean I created my back pain? Who would want to create pain like this? That's crazy!" The idea of personal responsibility in the creation of back pain may be hard to accept. But think what it actually means if we *do* create disease and pain. This is both good news and bad. The bad news is that we may have had some responsibility in creating this pain, but the good news is if we helped create pain, then we can help *un*-create it.

If it is still hard to accept that we can manifest disease or suffering in our bodies, that's all right. For now, try accepting at least half of this truth: that we can heal ourselves. Think about how a fractured bone knits itself, with some help of course from a physician who sets the bone and immobilizes it in a plaster cast. Once the bone is set, it "knows" how to grow back together. How do our bones "know?" The secret is what Norman Cousins, author of *Anatomy of an Illness,* calls the "physician who resides within," the body's own natural healing intelligence.

Cousins faced a debilitating and excruciatingly painful illness. Conventional medicine offered him little relief and hope for a cure. He knew of Hans Selye's ground-breaking work on stress, demonstrating a clear connection between stress, the negative emotions of fear, anger, and resentment, and subsequent illness. Cousins reasoned that if negative emotions could foster disease, then perhaps positive emotions could promote healing and health. He consequently moved out of his hospital room to a hotel, watched comedies, told jokes to everyone, and soon found out that ten minutes of deep "belly laughter" helped him sleep pain-free for two hours. Also he amazingly found that his blood sed rate, a measure of how ill he was, dropped five points after his first laughing session, and the drop held and was cumulative.

Now, we are *not* saying abandon your physician, rent funny videos and joke away back pain. (However, humor *is* important and is dealt with in a later chapter.) What's important about Cousins' discovery is the fact that he *chose* to take some initiative in his own healing process, rather than be a victim of illness. He chose to wake up the "physician within" and enlist him or her in the healing process.

It's all about choice. You are not a victim, unless you choose to be. A choice to take responsibility for healing means having power in the healing process. You can choose to work with your doctor and also use the healing suggestions herein to enhance and complement conventional medical treatment, and thus accelerate healing. You can choose to accept back pain as a message telling you to effect a change, rather than viewing it as something to suffer through. You can choose to be stuck with the hope of rescue always outside of your control. Our goal with this book is to eliminate suffering by offering healthier, more positive choices.

Doing something about pain makes you stronger, and less of a victim. Picking up this book shows a desire to do something to reduce pain. Working as a partner with a physician will dispel that sense of helplessness that can accompany chronic pain. Being in partnership with a doctor and the body's own natural "physician" can lift that cloud of victimhood, and speed healing. Hope and healing blossom with the choice to be proactive, instead of reactive. Norman Cousins' own journey proves positive emotions promote healing.

The first step in devictimizing back pain is to stop labeling it as "bad." Dr. Epstein again urges us to stop asking "why something that seems negative has happened to you." "The more you ask the question," he continues, "the more you will suffer and the more handcuffed you will feel." He also asserts that thinking "suffering is bad" itself perpetuates suffering—the very thing we are trying to overcome. He urges us to "accept what has happened as facts of [your] personal history" and to move on from there. This may seem like a tall order, to not call pain "bad." Of course, it's easy to label it bad—it hurts, it stops you from working, playing with your kids, and enjoying life. However, labeling it good or bad *doesn't* change the bad back. It still hurts. But labeling it bad and dwelling on the "badness" of it will increase suffer-

24

ing and not promote healing. When you no longer label it, space opens up to begin feeling better.

Clearly when faced with pain, you are at a point of choice. One choice leads to suffering and defeat. Another leads to growth and greater understanding. Neither choice is easy. But one choice has a more positive outcome and so it is worth the toughness it may take to walk that path. *Where pain leads is your choice.* This book aims to provide the courage, encouragement, and means to follow a path towards growth and wisdom. You are at the crossroads; choose *today* to walk towards a happier, fuller life.

Commitment to the Program

This program requires discipline and time. Unfortunately, clicking your heels or wiggling your nose will not result in an instant cure. However, if you are reading this book, then you are thinking about a deeper kind of healing.

The long form program may take up to $2^1/_2$ hours a day, not including the walking and recreational/social goals, and so perhaps you will think, "Where in the world will I find time to do all this? I'm busy. I work. I have a family. There's no extra time in my day!" Don't despair. Many of the activities can be combined with others (e.g. music with walking, or affirmations with breathing), and many of the acitivties are fun. But more importantly, consider how much time pain and discomfort take away from life now. How often in the last months have you missed work, or refused an invitation, or spent a whole day immobile in bed in pain? Think about a day when it took twice as long to do everything because of pain. You'll probably find that pain eats up quite a lot of time and life. That should provide some perspective on the time the long program requires, and demonstrate the value of the required time. What you do today *is* important. None of the programs outlined here can be done off and on. They will be most effective with consistency and discipline, and this requires commitment.

Now you're probably thinking, "Discipline? Commitment? Consistency? Those are scary words. It's going to be too hard. I don't think I can be disciplined and consistent enough, so maybe I'll just forget it." Don't close the book yet! For now, make the commitment to follow one of the programs for a week only. During this time, we think you'll be surprised by how good you'll feel. First, the decision to *do* something about pain and get involved in healing will lift your spirits. Second, the relaxation techniques will relieve a great deal of the stress you've no doubt been experiencing. Third, the pain-relief techniques really do work. We think that after a week the physical, mental, and emotional benefits will be apparent, and that in turn will drive the desire to be consistent and disciplined. The better you feel, the stronger the desire to continue; the longer and more consistently you stick with a program, the greater and more long-lasting the results.

Perhaps you might also think, "How can I take so much time every day *just* for me? Isn't that selfish?" A pain-free, healthier you is a gift to family, friends, and co-workers because they will all benefit from your greater health and happiness. You will be more available to family, more fun to be around for friends, and more productive and effective at work when pain-free, or pain has significantly been reduced. So, the gift of time each day to work on your well-being is not selfish at all.

Right now life is probably divided up into "good days," when you're more comfortable and thus more active, and "bad days," when discomfort truly interferes with life. Perhaps the ratio of pain-filled days to pain-free days leans heavily towards more pain-filled days. The aim of this program is of course to reverse this ratio, and eventually eliminate those bad days altogether.

A day may come in the first weeks of the program or perhaps even later, when you don't feel there's enough time to do the exercises, or make log entries. That's the time to remember that a bed unmade, a dish unwashed, a phone call unanswered, or a memo unwritten may not make a whole lot of difference in the long run. But the time devoted to healing *will* have an enormously positive effect. When the day comes that you just don't feel like doing an exercise, meditating, or checking off something in the log, try to keep things in proper perspective. Read this section again when discouraged or when you just can't seem to make the time to do the required activities. Finally, remember the healing work done that day *is* important in the greater scheme of things, and keep the commitment to the program.

However, if you have to skip a day, be gentle, do not beat yourself up for missing a day, and do not think you have failed. There are those days when life happens in the form of flat tires, lost keys, long meetings, traffic jams, and clogged drains, upsetting the day's whole plan. Suddenly it's nine in the evening and you haven't exercised. Just promise to do it the next day and know that this missed day does *not* negate all the good work accomplished so far. Gently reaffirm the commitment.

Time invested in dwelling on pain will yield a zero return, but time invested in the techniques outlined here, will yield a truly priceless return: pain relief. Today is the perfect time to begin. Commit to start the healing process and to keep it up as each new "today" dawns.

The Benefits of the Program in Addition to Pain Relief

This book's immediate aim is to reduce or relieve pain so that you can be active, go to work, and enjoy whatever activities you could once do or haven't done in awhile, because of back pain. But practicing the various techniques presented here with diligence will produce a far greater reward than immediate pain relief. With these techniques, the seeds of a richer, fuller, and more satisfying life are being planted.

One seed being planted that can be applied to other areas of life is the discipline and commitment required to follow the program. Perhaps you wish to stop smoking, lose weight, improve a golf swing, learn to play the piano, or take up fly fishing. These are all pursuits that require discipline and commitment.

Here is another valuable seed: *You* can do something about pain and illness, you do not have to be an unwitting and powerless victim of pain or anything or anyone else—ever again. It is empowering and comforting to know, for example, that you can use the acupressure techniques and your own fingers to relieve pain any time, any place; or that breathing can calm your mind and body whenever a bit of clarity and centering is needed in a stressful moment, or that you can shut the office door for fifteen minutes at lunch time to meditate and be totally refreshed and more productive for the afternoon; or that at the end of the day, you can relax deeply and sleep well without the aid of drugs, simply by hypnotizing yourself. These are all techniques you will learn with this book.

You will also find with self-hypnosis greater concentration and focus, and those will spill over into other areas of life. A teacher friend learned self-hypnosis, and found her teaching became much smoother and more focused. She would make detailed lesson plans, but when it came time to teach, she taught without notes and was fully present and engaged in the lesson, letting her creativity flow more, thus being a much more effective instructor. Learning to be still and in the moment, as required for hypnosis, has great value and can improve almost any area of life, from conducting board meetings to creating a perfect golf swing to interacting with family.

Also communicating with and opening up to the subconscious mind through self-hypnosis can make you more creative through direct access to the creative right side of the brain. Once you have opened up to this, a blossoming of creative energy may occur. If you've always wanted to write, paint, draw, build a new deck, or take up a new hobby, self-hypnosis may open up those channels, or more creative solutions to various problems at home or at work may emerge once the power of the subconscious mind is tapped.

Still another powerful seed being planted and nurtured in this program is the idea of *learning* from pain. It may sound Pollyanna-ish to say there is a silver lining to the pain, but remember you choose how to react to and perceive pain. Choosing to see it as empty, worthless suffering, a waste of valuable time, sends you down the victim's road discussed earlier, but learn to listen to and trust the body, and then take care of it. Learning from pain gives it positive meaning.

Once the mind has stretched around these new ideas, it can never quite go back to its former shape and size. Suffering or adversity will not be as daunting because you will have valuable skills to change the reaction to the bumps in the road of life. New choices, new varieties of hardy, resilient flowers will be planted in the garden of your life, along with new tools to keep that garden blooming.

What will be the gift of pain? What flowers will bloom in the garden you're planting by reading this book and following the programs outlined here? What fruit will you harvest from the lessons? This book shows how to plant the seeds, water them, and how to weed the garden. How diligently you nurture that garden is up to you. Following a program outlined here will yield a crop of hidden inner strengths and resources: a happier, more optimistic outlook on life, deeper understanding of yourself and others, greater creativity, hardier resiliency to life's ups and downs, and a stronger sense of destiny-shaping power.

Pain: A Useful Definition and its Transmission

Before we embark upon presenting an integrated pain management program, an understanding of pain and how it is transmitted to the brain is necessary.

All of us have felt pain. It can be burning, aching, piercing, gnawing, or electrical in nature. Indeed there are many other words to describe it. What exactly is pain? In *Mastering Pain,* by Dr. Richard A. Sternbach, pain is defined as "an unpleasant sensory and emotional experience associated with actual or potential tissue damage, or described in terms of such damage." Those with high pain tolerance can endure pain, while others with a low threshold experience pain in a deeply physical and emotional way.

There are two types of pain: acute and chronic pain. Acute pain is a positive type because it warns the body something is wrong. We have all experienced that sharp pain when we twist our ankle, sprain our back, or burn our hands. This type of pain is generally brief and while it may cause anxiety, our emotional state generally calms because we know it will soon get better. Chronic pain, what we are here concerned with, is a different phenomenon. Dr. Sternbach comments "The persistence of pain is called chronic pain. Chronic pain exists when an acute-pain problem has stabilized, that is, further healing is not likely to occur and there is not likely to be any change in the intensity of the pain itself. As a rule of thumb, any pain that persists for more than three to six months may be considered chronic." Sternbach further notes that chronic pain can vary in intensity from day to day, as well as with bodily position. In distinguishing acute from chronic pain, Sternbach explains that chronic pain is neither a warning signal, a symptom, nor a state that requires rest, but rather "chronic pain is a syndrome composed of a number of physical, emotional and behavioral changes which can convert otherwise healthy persons into invalids."

Why does it matter what type of pain it is, if it hurts nonetheless? The answer is important. Chronic pain is continuous pain that does not serve a useful purpose; in most cases the injury that caused acute pain has healed as much as it is going to heal, and rest is generally not required. What significance is this to you? It means that generally you can resume activities, including exercise, provided your physician approves. More importantly, it means that you can fully follow a program, provided your physician reviews and approves all elements of your chosen program.

Pain Transmission and the Gate Control Theory of Pain

Pain transmission is a complex process. Dr. Sternbach describes it as the transmission of injury signals to nerve fibers. In turn these signals are sent to other nerve fibers in the spinal cord, which then transmits pain signals electrically to the center of the brain. Pain, Sternbach points out, is not felt until the signal reaches the mid part of the brain, the thalamus. There, relays are made to the sensory cortex where we receive specific information about the pain. At the same time, the brain sends signals back down the spinal cord to dampen the injury signals.

In *The Book of Pain Relief*, Leon Chaitow explains the "gate theory." Because pain messages are carried along slow nerve fibers, by stimulating the faster nerve transmission fibers through vibration or acupuncture, we may be able to "shut the gate" to the messages "before and possibly after they enter the spinal cord for transmission to the brain." Chaitow gives us the following analogy of shutting the gate to pain: Pain signals initially open the gate into the central nervous system, but this gate can be partly or completely shut, either from the inside, through the influence of the mind, or from the outside by inhibitory mechanisms, such as acupuncture, touch or vibration. This is important to know, as it means human beings can control, with the mind or certain physical actions, pain messages to the brain, and have the power to release natural pain killers called endorphins, 700 more times powerful than morphine!

Brief Overview of Physical and Mental Means of Pain Control

All the pain reduction and relief techniques in this book fall into two general categories: physical and mental. Using these techniques "to close the gate to the pain message" is central to our program. You either use the mind to control pain, or move, stretch, and strengthen the body to achieve relief, or use both physical and mental means together. These concepts are briefly introduced below. In later chapters the various techniques are presented in detail, with precise instructions and illustrations.

Mental Means of Pain Control

Controlling the transmission of the pain message to the brain is key to pain relief, and we can control the message with our minds. The brain runs the autonomic nervous system, which is controlled by the subconscious mind. If you are crossing the street and a car appears headed straight for you, what happens? The autonomic nervous system immediately activates the flight-or-fight response. The heart beats faster, you become anxious and frightened, you may sweat and breathe hard, adrenaline is released, and muscles tense as the body instantaneously moves to take protective action.

Then that rush of energy needed to scoot out of harm's way surges through the body.

Just as the brain has the power to invoke this kind of powerful response, it also has, once properly trained, the ability to relieve and eliminate chronic pain. In later chapters, you will be taught how to activate "the physician that lives within" to enlist the body's healing intelligence and to release endorphins. Through pain distraction techniques, and through powerful relaxation techniques, you will learn how to reduce anxiety accompanying chronic pain, and different ways to perceive and react to pain so that suffering can be eliminated. Mental pain control works and is used daily by the most progressive pain management clinics throughout America. Just think, in a number of weeks you will be able to substantially relieve, if not eliminate back pain, by doing something as simple as taking three deep breaths and thinking "cool hands."

Briefly, what are these "mental" techniques? They are many and varied. As a preview, they are listed below:
• Positive Thinking and Affirmations
• Deep Breathing and Progressive Muscle Relaxation (although these are physical, learn them first as they are needed to master imagery and self-hypnosis)
• Self Hypnosis and Visualization or Imagery
• Humor and Music
• Meditation and Thought Stopping
• Helping Others
• Faith and Prayer
• Managing Stressors and Emotional Issues

Physical Means of Pain Relief

Just as pain can be controlled mentally, it can also be controlled physically. Bodily sensations such as touch, warmth, cold, or vibration can act as inhibitory mechanisms blocking or interfering with the transmission of pain signals. The physical means listed below primarily work on "the gate theory" and include:
• Ice and Heat
• Massage and Vibration
• Electrical Stimulation-TENS Units
• Salves and Ointments

Exercise helps to block pain signals through distraction and the release of endorphins. It also strengthens weak muscles and ligaments and stretches and lengthens contracted muscles, all helpful in preventing future pain. Included in the exercise section are:
• Warm-Up and Aerobic Exercises
• Strengthening and Stretching Exercises
• Back-specific Exercises
• Feldenkrais Movements
• Somatics Exercises and Walking

Various Eastern techniques can also be effective pain relievers. According to traditional Eastern medicine, the blockage and imbalance of "chi" is what causes illness and pain. Chi is defined as the vital life force energy that flows along meridians throughout each human body. The physical means of pain control that unblock the body's chi include:
• Reflexology and Acupressure
• Yoga and Tai-Chi
• Energy and Body Work

Once you have mastered the physical and mental means of pain relief, you should achieve considerable reduction in discomfort.

Some Likely Causes of Back Pain

If doctors cannot pinpoint the cause of back pain, it may be caused by one of eight, or a combination of eight, relatively common causes. Each cause is described below. Note references to relevant chapters on how to deal effectively with the causes under each description:

Chronic Muscle Contractions: The most probable common cause of chronic back pain is *involuntary, habituated* contractions of muscles associated with the back and legs, induced by stress, emotional factors, and/or continued contractions in reaction to ongoing pain. Based upon our own research, education in holistic health, in-depth discussions with medical and healing arts professionals and many who have cured their back pain, we have found this to be true for those who otherwise do not have a defined structural abnormality, documented disease, or serious injury. People with involuntary habituated contracted muscles have this problem in many areas of the back, buttocks, legs and tail bone. The muscles in these areas are no longer subject to control. Those who have obtained partial or full pain relief have learned how to *voluntarily* control their contracted muscles and have also recognized and possibly resolved stressful and emotional issues causing the tension.

Stress and unrecognized/unresolved emotional issues, generally thought of as psychological, can have a real, physical effect on the body, affecting muscles in a number of ways. These issues can cause contraction of abdominal muscles and all other muscles associated with tucking ourselves into a ball, or muscles associated with arching the back. Unfortunately, these contractions can become involuntary. Human beings are not necessarily programmed for the level of stress in modern, industrial society. Indeed, in less developed non-industrial societies, where stress is at a reduced level, painful backs are reported less often. In our current stressful times, individuals often have constantly tense involuntarily contracted leg, buttock, and lower and upper back muscles. Pain results from the muscles' inability to fully relax, as well as the resulting build up of lactic acid. The situation snowballs when a person rests too much and does not exercise due to fear of renewed pain, thereby aggravating the condition resulting in further contractions. Fortunately, this habituated state of involuntary muscle contractions can be altered.

Chronic pain patients who have achieved significant relief have two main characteristics: First, from a mental standpoint, they have recognized and resolved, or learned to live with, stressors and emotional issues in their lives. Second, through a designed exercise program, they have regained conscious control over their problem muscles. Simply put, they have learned to relax their minds and muscles and have *unlearned* habituated contractions, thus eliminating a state of chronic muscle tension.

A number of chapters focus on these issues. Chapters 16-20 cover The Exercise Program, Feldenkrais Movement Therapy, Somatics Movement Therapy, Proper Posture, Yoga and Tai Chi. Additionally, these chapters will help identify contracted muscles and loosen them through stretching and strengthening. The guidelines and journalizing program in Chapter 3, will help you recognize and cope with stress and emotional issues. Professional help of a psychologist or psychiatrist may also be needed. Do not misunderstand us. The pain is real, it is a chronic disease, and it is not in your head. One way to treat it may be from the viewpoint of continued habituated muscle contractions. You do not have to learn to live with it. In Chapter 27 you will learn about nutritional supplements, vitamins, and amino acids that can also help loosen tense muscles.

The various physical and mental means herein are the tools to deal with the contractions and their underlying causes. The following sections detail the various muscles which commonly contract under stressful conditions. The key to managing or possibly eliminating chronic pain lies in the ability to reduce stress, ensuring that these muscles, once loosened, will remain uncontracted.

Tight Hamstring Muscles: Tight hamstring muscles are a major cause of back pain. Here is a simple test for tight hamstring muscles. Lie on the back with the legs straight out on the floor. Slowly lift the right leg up, keeping the leg as straight as possible. If you can only get the leg up to a 30-50 degree angle, without strain in the calf or back of the thigh, you have tight hamstring muscles. If raising the leg induces pain in the back or sharp shooting pain down the leg, this may not be a result of tight hamstrings; you may have a disc problem and should discuss this with a doctor before commencing the program. If there is simply strain in the calf or thigh upon raising the leg, there is a good chance your back pain may be caused by tight hamstring muscles. Try the same test on the left leg. In Chapter 16 there are exercises for stretching the hamstrings, and in Chapter 26 there are specific touch techniques for loosening these muscles.

Weak Stomach Muscles: Weak stomach muscles are also a prime culprit in back pain. Weak stomach muscles are apparent if you've ever tried to do sit ups and ended up with trembling abdominals and a red face. Also if the belly is protruding, that may also be a sign of weak abdominals. Strong stomach muscles are very important because they support the back. Chapter 16 gives detailed instructions for abdominal strengthening exercises.

Tight Psoas Muscles: A tightened or de-energized psoas muscle is a major cause of back pain. This muscle starts in the groin, goes under the butt, and attaches to the spine from approximately the mid-back through the lower back (See the muscle chart in Chapter 26). A very effective exercise to loosen the psoas muscle is the hip-flexor stretch in Chapter 16.

Tight Leg Muscles: Other tight leg muscles, including the quadriceps (muscles on the front of the thighs), facsia lata (muscles on the outside of thighs), piriformis (deep muscle near facsia lata) and the calf muscles (on the back of the lower legs), (See chart in Chapter 26) as well as tight hamstrings, can also be the cause of back pain. *All these muscles need to be spasm free and flexible.* Follow the instructions in Chapter 16 for the quadriceps stretch, standing side stretch, prone extension, and calf stretch, and directions in Chapter 26 for stretching

the piriformis muscle. Piriformis syndrome is a major cause of back pain.
Improper Posture, Poor Sitting, Standing and Walking Habits: A major cause of back pain relates to improper posture. Compare your sitting, standing and walking postures with those discussed in Chapter 19 on proper posture. Correcting and maintaining proper sitting, standing, and walking postures should reduce pain levels.

Muscle Imbalances: Imbalances in major muscle groups of the back and legs are often a leading cause of back pain. For example, if the muscles on the right side of the back are very tight and those on the left are weak, muscles on the right compensate for those on the left, and major muscle imbalances occur. The exercises in chapters 16-18 should help restore muscle balance.

Improper Foot Support: Improper shoes mean poor foot support, and studies have shown this can cause imbalances affecting the back. Weak and painful arches, improper heel support, or one leg shorter than the other, may generate severe back pain. We recommend seeing a podiatrist who will check for improper foot support and short-leg syndrome, and will be able to prescribe orthotics, or shoe inserts for proper support. Orthotics are often covered by insurance. If you do not want to visit a podiatrist, try drugstore shoe inserts. If they offer relief, you're headed in the right direction and should consult a podiatrist. Short-leg syndrome can be adjusted with a shoe lift for the affected leg.

Object of the Program: A Summing Up

Simply put, the object of the program is to reduce or eliminate chronic back pain. Chaitow, in *The Book of Pain Relief*, concludes that there are three elements to pain relief: 1. understanding the pain; 2. anxiety reduction; and 3. distraction.

We would add an important fourth to the list: blocking pain signals through mental and physical means. The methodologies presented here teach how to distract yourself from the pain through exercise and other physical and mental activities, how to reduce anxiety levels through relaxation techniques, and most important, physical and mental means that block pain signals and stimulate endorphin production. Our program will transform your negative attitude towards pain.

Methodology of the Program

The methodology of the program is simple. It requires participation in a goal setting and accomplishment program using a daily log form. You must commit to various attitudinal, social, recreational, vocational, exercise, relaxation, pain management, pain flare-up, and weight loss, vitamin and supplement goals, instituted by yourself. We will set forth three recommended programs: the long form, the short form, and the design-your-own. However, you may choose from many pain relief techniques. The long program may take up to three hours per day, but should help tremendously. The short program is included for those who cannot meet the time demands of the long program. Moreover, much of it will be fun, challenging, and will improve the quality of life. The design-your-own program contains recommendations as to the minimum requirements for a sound pain management program. To save time, elements such as humor with walking may be combined. Just think how much better off you will be by investing time in these programs rather than worrying about on-going pain.

The Equipment

The scope of our program is extremely broad. Full participation and success will require the use of certain equipment. After reading the foregoing sections, the importance of equipment to enhance the program's effectiveness should be apparent. First we list the required equipment and then the recommended, but optional equipment. Recommendations for highly effective products will also be made in relevant chapters as well as in this section.

Required Equipment:

• Exercise Mat: A firm, yet soft exercise mat is required. Physical exercise is a key ingredient in relieving pain, but carpet or hard floor may increase pain. Invest in a comfortable mat as you will need it for the physical exercises and also for many mental means of pain relief such as meditating and deep breathing, which may require that you lie on the floor.

• Light Weights: Two sets of weights, 3 lb. and 5 lb. for each set, are essential for strengthening exercises. The 3-lb. set, (1.5 lb. for each hand) will be used to strengthen back muscles. The 5-lb. set should be structured so each 2.5-lb. weight can be attached to feet to strengthen leg muscles.

• Three-Ring Binder, File Separators and Paper: You will need a three-ring binder to store weekly program log forms and any other useful material you find. Keeping track of what you do each day will help you to comply with the program, and afford a sense of accomplishment. The notebook will also store the Daily Pain Tracking Journal and Weekly Summary forms. We suggest keeping records tracking pain reduction progress, as well as writing down good jokes and visualization exercises. It is important to note critical insights so they don't just float in and out of the mind altogether—you may forget a valuable insight that might help later. A log of successful pain reducing techniques discovered in readings or in speaking to others, and helpful pamphlets and magazine articles should also be stored in this binder.

• Library Card: The local library contains a treasure trove of materials on and for pain relief. Just think about all those books on humor sitting on the shelf—humor that will stimulate endorphins and relieve pain. Do not forget that many libraries have extensive cassette or CD collections ranging from comedy to music. Many libraries in big cities also lend video tapes.

• A Good Pair Of Walking Shoes: Walking is an important form of exercise. Shoes with good support are a must. Invest some money here; it is worth it.

• A Moist Heating Pad and Ice Packs: Moist heat from an adjustable heating pad can quickly uncontract your muscles. Ice packs can also be a good pain reliever. You probably have each of these items anyway, but if not, please acquire them. You might be slightly sore in the beginning from some of the exercises and moist heat soothes those aching muscles.

• *Healing Back Pain—The Mind Body Connection* by Dr. John Sarno: This book is necessary for the program in Chapter 3.

Recommended Items:

The following are not required but will greatly assist you in accomplishing certain elements of the program:

• Regular CD Player With Remote: The remote is useful as we will ask you to pause the CD during the exercise programs. A portable player with headphones will enable you to listen to the CDs in private while away from home without disturbing others. (As noted previously, the CDs are available from the authors, see Appendix E for ordering information.).

• Exercise Equipment or an Exercise Video That Will Make You Sweat: You will be need to warm the muscles up through some form of aerobic conditioning. An electric treadmill is best. But since they can be expensive, consider a used one or look for a manual treadmill. If that is too expensive, look for an non-electric exercise bike. A decent one can be purchased for under $100.

Whatever you choose, get something that induces a sweat in a 10 to 20 minute aerobic workout. Gentle workouts on video exercise tapes can serve the same purpose.

• A Portable Jacuzzi or Spa: Warm swirling water is a powerful pain reliever and muscle relaxant. There are inexpensive portable units you can place in the bathtub. A hot tub that would be wonderful, but certainly not required.

• A Good Vibrator or Massager: At a local drug store, these range in price from $15 to $100. Get what feels good. Electric is fine, but one that includes rechargeable batteries can be taken anywhere. Continuous vibrational massage loosens tight muscles and relieves pain.

• Infrared Heat: An infrared heating device provides deep penetrating heat and is an effective pain reliever.

• A VCR That Records and A Cable Hookup: VCRs are inexpensive today. They are good pain relievers, for they can record great comedy, dramas and music videos. A wealth of comedy is aired on cable TV 24 hours a day.

• A Mind Machine: In Chapter 14 mind machines are discussed. They are excellent tools for relaxation and reprogramming the brain. While somewhat expensive, they can quickly place your brain in a theta state, ideal for relaxation and learning and pain relief.

• Portable Cassette Player: A battery powered Walkman is excellent for listening to relaxation music or comedy. Music while walking or meditating enhances the experience. You may also want to purchase a cassette player to record tapes or record comedy or music off TV or radio.

• Books, Audio CDs, Cassettes and Video Tapes: Throughout the text we make references to excellent books, audio CDs, audio cassette tapes and video tapes. You may wish to purchase some of these.

• The Sacro-Wedgy: A small, inexpensive, almost doorstop-shaped, rubber wedge that is placed under the tailbone while you are lying on the floor. Lying on it for 20 minutes is highly effective for relaxing the hips and lower back. It can be ordered from B & B Marketing, (800) 737-9295.

• The Theracane: This is a 2-foot long, hard plastic cane-like device with 6 knobs in various positions along its surface. It can be used to massage hard-to-reach acupressure points all over the body, and should be available in any back care store, medical device or physical therapy supply house.

• Back Massager With Heat: The Homedics Back Pleaser Ultra is a seat pad with a high back that contains five massage motors and heating elements throughout the pad. It can be plugged in and used at home, but it also has an adaptor that allows you to use it in the car. It is highly effective for loosening tight back and hamstring muscles.

• Anything that is Comforting and Calming: It's your choice here, those extras that calm, relax, or otherwise nurture. These could range from incense to candles, to pillows, to chamomile tea, to an aromatherapy scent diffuser or a sound machine for soothing surrounding sounds of a rainforest or mountain stream. Relaxation relieves anxiety and tension, loosening tight muscles.

CHAPTER 2

GOAL SETTING AND ACCOMPLISHMENT: THE KEY TO ENHANCING YOUR LIFE AND RELIEVING PAIN

Introduction

THE SETTING AND ACCOMPLISHMENT OF GOALS are the foundation of our program, a strong focus of the Stanford Medical Center's Pain Management program, and what enabled author Miller to resume his life in full after suffering chronic back pain. Goals motivate you to get better and determine how you desire to live. In his book, *Mastering Pain*, Dr. Richard Sternbach notes that "you need to have goals as reasons for overcoming your pain," and that having specific goals is the reason one "copes with pain." The focus shifts away from pain when you set and accomplish goals.

Goal Setting

Setting goals is required in the following areas:
- positive thinking activities
- vocational, social and recreational activities
- pain management skills
- pain flare-up control skills
- utilization of health care resources
- weight control, vitamins, supplements and nutrition

Set realistic, reachable goals so that you have the confidence to achieve the targeted activities on a weekly or daily basis. While we will make certain recommendations in these areas, the specific goals will be your choice. However, failure to set goals in each category will impede progress.

Before beginning, be sure to discuss chosen goals with your physician, especially those of exercise, weight control and nutrition. Also ask about the role pain medications may have as a complement to techniques from this book.

Positive Thinking Activities

Positive thinking is essential to the success of a pain relief program. Because it is so important, we have devoted a whole chapter to it and recommend *daily* goals in this area to make it an ongoing part of the pain management program. The activities that foster positive thinking are presented in detail in Chapter 4, but in brief they consist of the following:

• Identifying and stopping negative thoughts
• Replacing negative thoughts with more positive ones
• Journaling (Keeping a daily journal)
• Affirmations

Imagery and self-hypnosis, detailed in Chapters 5 and 6, promote positive thinking as well and should also be daily goals.

Vocational Goal Activities

Work goals are important. Vocational activities can mean work for wages, volunteer work or even study. Dr. Sternbach, in *Mastering Pain*, states that having work goals is important because "it may provide additional income; it gives...pride in accomplishment and in being able to overcome a handicap; it keeps (people)...busy and less likely to get in poor mental and physical condition; and it keeps (people's)...minds off the pain so it is not noticed as much."

If you are currently working in a chosen vocation/profession, set specific goals. Explore special projects or certain achievements. If you can no longer physically handle the work in a previous vocation/profession due to back injury or chronic pain, consider alternative vocations. Seek help from professional vocational rehabilitation counselors.

If you do not or cannot work full or part time, consider volunteering in the community to assist others. Helping others is a very powerful pain relieving technique. Volunteer in areas which interest you. (See the Chapter 9 on Connecting With Others for suggestions about where to volunteer.) If you do not want to volunteer, set study goals. Consider going back to school to gain proficiency in a personally interesting field. It will get the mind off pain and provide an objective to strive for.

Social Activities

Contact with other human beings significantly reduces pain levels, but understandably, those in chronic pain often become irritable and withdrawn. Dr.

Sternbach states that increasing social relationships is "comforting"and distracts from pain. We suggest establishing social goals such as a movie, a ball game, lunch with co-workers, or dinner with friends. Yes, even increasing sexual activity with a spouse or partner is appropriate. These activities lift the spirits and reduce discomfort.

Recreational Activities

Fun is distracting, and more importantly, releases endorphins. Indeed, fun puts a more positive spin on life, shifting your attitude from despair to hope and enthusiasm. Many of you will say, "I can no longer do what I used to do for fun." That might be true, but think about the scores of activities you *can* do. While long bike rides or vigorous hikes may not be possible now, a number of other activities are possible, and those you did before can certainly be done in moderation. Expand your interests in previously unexplored areas. Set specific recreational goals on a daily basis: exercise, sports, hobbies, or even fun mental activities such as watching comedy on TV or becoming proficient in computers. Take two 30-minute walks a day, a weekend bike ride, catch up on movies, or pursue a favorite hobby. Make sure some of these outings involve moving. Dr. Sternbach advises that fun gives you something to look forward to, the pleasure of anticipation, and "time out from pain," because with absorption in an activity, discomfort is "not noticed as much, or doesn't seem to bother as much."

Pain Management Goals

We will recommend certain physical and mental means of pain control that are very effective, but we present more than you will likely use. Goals in this area are very important and essential to successful pain reduction. Read the entire book *before* choosing any pain management goals.

For pain management, we recommend selecting a number of physical means of pain control, one of which must be an exercise program, and some mental means of pain control, one of which must be guided imagery. Exercise and imagery must be done on a daily basis. Remember, if any of the recommended techniques are not effective, there is a wide variety of others to choose from. The selection should also be discussed with your physician.

Pain Flare-Up Control Skills

Pain flare-ups are frightening and frustrating, so it is important to know which means of pain control will help most immediately and effectively. What will help most is highly individualized and only you know what will work. We suggest having at least two readily-available mental and physical methods of pain control to get through a crisis. Medicine may be appropriate, but quick-acting distractions such as a particular exercise, humor, music, deep breathing, or stretching can help a great deal and might be better than medication. The chapters on mental and physical means of pain control offer concrete ways to deal with a flare-up. A plan is important because knowing you have it can reduce the crisis anxiety.

Utilization of Health Care Resources

Following your physician's treatment plan is essential. You may say, "Nothing is working, so why should I listen to the doctor who has not cured me?" When discussing goal setting and accomplishment with your physician, he/she will no doubt have suggestions and may prescribe pain killing medication. Follow your doctor's orders and take medication as prescribed. On the other hand, since your condition is chronic, unless there has been a noticeable change in the condition there is no need to run from doctor to doctor or to the emergency room with each flare up. Sample contracts for each program are at the end of Chapter 28, and daily entries on each indicate compliance with doctor's or physical therapist's instructions, including taking medications. Other spaces indicate that you are not going to the emergency room or doctorís office unless truly necessary.

Weight Control, Vitamins, Supplements & Nutrition

Weight control, vitamins, herbs and nutrition are discussed later as a significant means of pain control. Weight control is critical because the less weight the back has to support the better, and certain vitamins, supplements and herbs have strong pain killing abilities. Make goal choices from our recommendations, but discuss them with your physician as they may conflict with prescribed medications. A healthy diet means a stronger body and better muscle tone.

The Pain Management Contract and Sample Program

In Chapter 28 three different contracts detail what we recommend. Whichever program you choose, bear in mind this is a contract with yourself that you will want to keep, for one week at a time. Under the goal activities column, list the specific activities you wish to accomplish. Under the frequency column, note frequency of the chosen activity per week. Under the day and date column, check off each goal activity as it is completed. To make record keeping easier, have the contract with you at all times. Following the program in this manner will be satisfying and help you take control of the pain, while at the same time enriching your life. Remember, you can change the goals any time. You are in control.

The Daily "To Do" List

As an additional aid to ensure compliance with the program, we recommend setting up a daily "to do" list. We have provided a chart for you to photocopy and use to plan and track your compliance on a daily basis. Once an item is done, check off the goal on the "to do" list and on the contract. There is also space on the chart for you to note what worked best for you on a particular day so that you can begin to determine which techniques will work best in case of a flare-up.

Discipline and organization are essential. Remember, the busier you are, the better the pain relief. At a minimum the pain will lessen and greater reduction will follow, provided you stay with the chosen program and remain busy.

DAILY TO DO LIST

Day and Date_____

Time of Day	Attitude, Recreational, Social, Vocational, Activities	Mental & Physical Means of Pain Management
Morning		
Afternoon		
Evening		
Night		

What Worked Best for Me Today?

Physical Means	Mental Means

CHAPTER 3

THE ROLE OF STRESS AND EMOTIONS IN CHRONIC BACK PAIN

Introduction

WHILE THIS CHAPTER IS RELATIVELY SHORT, it is one of the most important in the book. Please read it carefully. As noted in the opening chapter, the cause of most chronic back pain is involuntary habitually-contracted muscles induced by stress, emotional issues, and an ongoing reaction to the pain. The professionals treating author Miller at Stanford concurred with this explanation. The goal of this chapter is to show how stress and emotional issues can cause back pain, provide tools to identify and resolve these issues, as well as to share how one individual cured emotionally-induced chronic back pain.

How Can Stress and Emotional Issues Result in Back Pain?

Hundreds of research studies and books have chronicled the bodily effects of stress, ranging from rapid heartbeat to cool hands to breathing pattern changes. One of the most common physiological effects is the tightening of muscles in the lower back, pelvic area, and legs, often resulting from the fight-or-flight response, dating from prehistory when humans encountered life-threatening situations on a daily basis. When we are faced with immediate danger, various hormones rush into the bloodstream to give us either the will and strength to stand and fight, or the surge of muscle power we may need to escape. Although nowadays most of us do not face beasts of prey, the fight-or-flight response is still triggered when we encounter stressful, but not necessarily life-threatening, situations such as heavy traffic, pressure at work, home or school, or an argument with a spouse or partner. In our fast-paced society, we frequently face tremendous pressures from financial, job- and family-related demands on our time and energy. In response to these modern-day pressures, the hormones that helped us escape from a woolly mammoth thousands of years ago flood our bloodstream, causing muscles to tighten and hearts to race. The real trouble begins when muscles remain contracted long after the stressful circumstances pass.

How does this relate to chronic back pain? Pain may be drastically reduced by identifying the stressors and the emotional reactions to them, and understanding how these stressors affect muscle systems. *Most important, however, to the success of a pain management program is to take action for the effective elimination or resolution of the issues and circumstances that cause tense muscles.*

Identifying Stressors and Emotional Issues

Each of us is different; what unnerves you may not affect someone else. Be extremely honest in recognizing what stressors exist in your life. Indeed, the help of a professional psychologist or psychiatrist may be necessary. We recommend, that in consultation with a physician or therapist, establishing a journal that lists the stressors, the emotional issues associated with them, a plan to resolve them, and noting if pain levels increase due to the identified stressor. We have included a Daily Pain Tracking Journal form and a Weekly Summary to help you track the kinds of events (both physical and non-physical) that cause stress and result in increases in pain. By tracking pain levels on a daily basis you can begin to see patterns and then take action to change the patterns. But first, of course, you must be able to identify them.

We are all probably aware of the kinds of events and circumstances that cause major stresses in our lives: death of a family member, divorce, employment termination, or a major illness or injury. These of course result in a variety of emotions such as grief, anger, fear, resentment, or despair.

There are also the more day-to-day kinds of stresses we often face: computer crashes, arguments with spouses, children, neighbors, or co-workers, conflicts with bosses, dealing with commute traffic or not catching an important flight, missing a meeting, and all the demands of everyday life in the late 20th century. These too can result in the negative emotions of anger, fear, frustration, and resentment, and result in raised pain levels. These types of stressors are referred to as non-physical stressors.

Physical stressors, such as poor posture, sitting slumped over, sitting for extended periods of time, over exercising, stretching while muscles are cold, lifting improperly etc. can result in back pain. See Chapter 19 for a discussion of proper physical form.

Below is a typical entry in the *Daily Pain Tracking Journal.* On your pain management contract the process is referred to as journaling.

Time of Day	Stressor?		Pain Level? 1-low to 5-intense	Emotional Reaction (name it: anger, fear, resentment, despair, etc.)
	Physical (e.g., sitting too long)	Non-Physical (conflict at work)		
Morning	Sat slumped over at work	Argument with wife prior to work	1-2-3-4-5	Anger and frustration with wife

There is space on this form for you to monitor your pain levels and non-physical and physical stressors morning, afternoon, evening, and night. Complete the journal daily.

A typical entry on the Weekly Summary might look like this:

Worst day this week? Monday
Highest pain level that day? 4
Triggering stressor? Argument with wife.
Emotion? Anger and frustration.
How can I resolve this issue? (action plan) Consider wife's views carefully and count to ten before screaming at her.

Photocopy the appropriate number of forms and use them on a daily and weekly basis to track pain levels and stressors to determine a pattern and then think how you can resolve, change, or at least decrease the stressors.

For those in continual or intermittent back pain, *the pain itself* can be a true stressor. Fear, hopelessness, and anxiety are ever present, and muscles can get even tighter. We hope, however, the programs in this book will turn this stressor around. Remember that the mind is the most powerful force to control, manage, and eliminate chronic pain. Your goals relative to this chapter are to identify the stressors and emotional issues that may contribute to or cause the muscle contractions. We suggest some positive self talk to affirm that you will not let stressors or the associated emotions cause the muscles to contract.

An affirmation/response activity is another interesting method that we have personally used to identify the stressors possibly involved in back pain. You can do it alone or with a friend. The basic technique is as follows: State out loud, "My back is pain-free." Then immediately write down or have your friend write down the first thought that comes to mind. Keep repeating "My back is pain free" and writing the response down until no new responses enter your mind. The last new response to the repeated statement is probably the very issue that is bothering you.

Program To Cure Chronic Back Pain Associated With Emotional Issues
Throughout the literature and on the Internet we have heard positive words about an excellent book entitled *Healing Back Pain: The Mind-Body Connection* by Dr. John Sarno. Many people asserted that the principles in this book successfully resolved their back pain. We have read the book and recommend it highly, as it deals with emotional issues relative to back pain. While on the Internet we had the good fortune to meet an individual who developed a program based on this book, resulting in a pain-free back after over two years of debilitating pain. As you may wish to try it, the steps in his program are presented below:

1. Read *Healing Back Pain: The Mind-Body Connection* from cover to cover.

2. Read 30 pages of the book daily and think about how its concepts apply to your personal situation. Focus on the fact that the people mentioned had real back problems and were cured.

3. After finishing the book, reading 30 pages a day, start reading it again the next day. Read it continuously for a month.

4. Spend a minimum of 30 minutes a day, preferably 15 minutes in the morning and 15 minutes in the evening, thinking about what is bothering you and what might be so troubling as to cause physical problems. Be specific about the nature of the problem. Write lists or keep a journal. Pay close attention to

all life areas, noting both obvious problems and possible hidden ones. Consider real and imagined items as well. Prime issues could be work or school problems, financial pressures, family responsibilities, relationships with spouses, significant others, parents or children, or any other important issue.

After identifying the problems, classify them into two groups: those that you can do something about and those that are *beyond your control* to change. Be realistic about what category each problem fits into. For those that you can do something about, develop an action plan to tackle them and immediately get to work. Do everything possible to correct the problems. For those that you have no control over, tell yourself while they are annoying, you must accept them; but you *will not* let them cause any more back pain. Seriously think about who you are and what you are like--what *is* it within your personality that allows problems to create pain. Be honest in this process.

5. Keep the cure process in mind all the time and keep reminding yourself of the process.

6. Whenever a problem comes up, think, "Okay I do not like that, but I am not going to let that go to my back and cause me pain."

7. Whenever the pain occurs, ask what is going on that may be triggering discomfort.

8. After working on these steps for 3-4 weeks, start taking small steps to test progress. Go slowly, but notice if the pain is less. Build on small steps, but even the slightest improvement shows that the process is working.

9. Be persistent and do not give up.

DAILY PAIN TRACKING JOURNAL

Day and Date_____

Time of Day	Stressor		Pain Level 1-low to 5-intense	Emotional Reaction (name it: anger, fear, resentment, despair, etc.)
	Physical (e.g., sitting too long)	**Non-physical** (e.g., conflict with co-worker)		
Morning			1-2-3-4-5	
Afternoon			1-2-3-4-5	
Evening			1-2-3-4-5	
Night			1-2-3-4-5	

WEEKLY SUMMARY OF DAILY PAIN TRACKING JOURNAL

Use this chart to summarize and note any patterns and connections between stressors and pain levels you see in reviewing the *Daily Plan Tracking Journal*. Then make plans to resolve the issues that cause pain levels to rise.

Week of_____

Worst Day This Week	**Worst Time of Day This Week**
Highest Pain Level That Day	**Highest Pain Level at That Time**
Triggering Stressor	**Triggering Stressor**
Emotion	**Emotion**
How Can I Resolve This Issue? (action plan)	**How Can I Resolve This Issue?** (action plan)

Best Day This Week	**Pain Level**
Lack of Physical Stressors?	
Lack of Non-Physical Stressors	
Emotions	
What I Learned This Week by Observing My Pain Levels in Response to Stressors	

CHAPTER 4

POSITIVE THINKING: CHANGE YOUR MIND, CHANGE YOUR LIFE

WE HAVE TOUCHED BRIEFLY on the issue of changing your experience by changing your thoughts, and in this section we will discuss in greater detail the value of positive thinking to the healing process. This information serves as a theoretical foundation for what follows in the chapters on self-hypnosis and imagery, and offers concrete ways to alter thinking patterns with various techniques including thought stopping and affirmations.

What Is It?

First of all, let us define negative thinking before we discuss positive thinking. The authors of the *Chronic Pain Control Workbook* note there are eight types of negative thinking:

• Blaming: This means blaming either others or yourself for the chronic pain situation.

• Shoulds: Should statements, such as "I should be better by a certain time," create negative and often impossible expectations. Statements such as, "My spouse should offer me more support or sympathy for my condition," also create negative expectations for others.

• Polarized Thinking: This is black and white, all-or-nothing thinking. Negative thoughts that may occur during a relapse are most damaging, as you may then think the pain control program is no good and should be abandoned.

• Catastrophizing: This entails imagining the worst possible outcome of what may be a tiny set-back. For example, the *Workbook* views "what if" statements as illustrative of this type of thinking. Typical of these kinds of statements might be, "What if my pain never gets better, and I have to live like an invalid for the rest of my life and my spouse leaves me and I lose my job and my house and end up in a wheelchair?"

• Control Fallacies: Here you may see your chronic pain situation as "externally controlled" by others. Conversely, you may impose "internal controls," making yourself entirely responsible for the pain.

• Emotional Reasoning: Here *feelings* become reality. Feelings at a given moment, especially during a pain flare-up, seem so real that you invest a lot of emotional energy on them. The *Workbook* notes, if one day you feel hopeless, thinking the pain will never stop, then you will come to believe it will never stop. "The strength of the feelings creates conviction, but things may later seem very different as the emotional storm dies down."

• Filtering: This means focusing only on one thing and failing to see positive elements. Indeed the pain becomes worse because it is the entire focus. One patient became so obsessed with the fear of another back attack, that she "filtered out her doctor's advice on prevention and exercise."

• Entitlement Fallacy: Again thinking in absolutes, believing you are entitled to a pain free existence, or life is just unfair. The world owes you!

All of us at one time or another have had thoughts such as these. Someone in pain may frequently think, "I will never get better," or "I have no control over the pain," or "I can't take another minute of this damn pain!" These kinds of thoughts give rise to fear, fear tenses muscles, and tight muscles intensify pain. Pain then gives rise to more negative thoughts. It is a vicious cycle. If your thinking falls into any of the above eight patterns, whether occasionally or habitually, this chapter will be most useful.

Positive thinking does not mean ignoring a problem, burying your head in the sand to escape, glossing over pain, pretending it's not there, or grinning and bearing pain. Positive thinking is simply the decision to look at and think about a situation from a different angle, with patience and compassion and without being judgmental.

Looking at the current situation with patience allows you to be happy with any healing progress, and if you've made none (or what you *think* is none), it still allows you to say, "Okay, I can wait. I can be patient enough to work on this even if it takes some time." In the midst of pain, it may seem eternal, but remember that all things pass and nothing lasts forever. Patience to deal with the present moment of pain comes with an open mind. Impatience, wanting healing *now*, blocks energy, focuses thinking on the pain, and increases suffering. Patience fosters hope, and hope opens up the way for the energy flow of change and healing.

Viewing the situation without judgment opens space to just *be*. As noted earlier, back pain is neither good nor bad--it just is. Judgment keeps you stuck in pain because judging requires *focusing* on the pain. With patience and non-judgment you are more likely to say, "My back *can* be better." "Can," unlike "should" allows room for possibilities and focuses on the positive end result. Patience, without judgment, allows you to be more compassionate. Compassion and gentleness relieve suffering. Gently remind yourself that you are working on healing and you are getting stronger and better.

Positive thinking is simply the decision to shift from "I can't stand one more day of pain," to "I can do this one day at a time," from "My back should be better" to "My back can be better," and from "Life is awful because I'm in pain and can't do what I want to do," to "I'm in pain and some things are hard for me *now*, but I am working on getting better."

Why Does It Work?

There are three basic principles that power positive thinking:
• The universe is energy.
• Thoughts can produce visible, tangible results though they themselves are invisible and intangible.
• What you think about all the time is what grows in your life.

Everything in the universe is energy. This book is energy of a dense, slow-moving kind. The chair you're sitting on now is energy of the same type as the book. Our thoughts are also energy. Though obviously not of the same density as this book, thoughts are very real even though we cannot touch them as we can touch this book or your chair. However, this book *began* as a thought and is now a physical reality you can see, touch, and read! Since thoughts are energy, it's important then to direct the thought energy towards the goal of pain relief and health.

Thoughts can have a measurable physical effect on the body. Think of someone scraping his nails across a blackboard and goose bumps rise even though it's "just a thought." Think about a favorite food whether it's pizza, roast beef, or a hot fudge sundae, and your mouth waters.

Negative thoughts adversely affect the physical state and can dramatically increase anxiety and pain levels. Imagine now a time when you were really angry. Blood pressure and heart rate may increase though you're "only thinking." Fear of the dentist, makes the mere *thought* of a dental appointment bring on sweaty palms and a fluttery stomach. Thus it is clear that nonphysical thoughts can have a physical effect, therefore think what effect negative thoughts produce on the body, including the back muscles.

Because thoughts are energy, what we think about all the time is what tends to grow in our lives. That is why it's important to stop letting thoughts of pain fill the mind day after day. Obsessing about pain, thinking about it all the time, talking about it to everyone within earshot, makes the pain the focus of your life, and it grows! How much better to fill the mind with thoughts of well-being. Then well-being is what will grow.

How Do You Do It?

Self-hypnosis and imagery, outlined in upcoming chapters, are excellent ways to incorporate positive thinking. However, there are many other things to do on a day-to-day basis to become a more positive-thinking person, not just around pain, but in general. The techniques below are provided to help you become more optimistic about reducing pain and healing, but they can also be applied to any area of life in which a change is desired.

The following suggestions come from the book, *You Can't Afford the Luxury of a Negative Thought,* by Peter McWilliams, an excellent source for people who want to become positive thinkers.

Thought Monitoring: To start, for one day monitor the negative thoughts and words used to describe pain. Do you say things like, "My back is killing me today?" Just gently notice what kind of language you use to talk about pain to yourself and to others. Notice what kinds of thoughts come up with pain.

Pause After a Negative Thought: After monitoring negative words and thoughts for some time, then the next step is to pause before speaking negatively. When a negative thought comes up, stop and think about something else--something pleasant. Keep a list of pleasant or uplifting thoughts close at hand for these times. (See the section in this chapter on affirmations for ideas in this area.) Be gentle, but allow the time between the negative thought and its vocal expression to grow in length.

Negative Thought-Free Time: Set times during the day for *no* negative thoughts. Start with a few minutes and build up to longer and longer periods. Focus on only good thoughts, on any progress, on anything good happening right now.

Just Say No: If a negative thought comes into the mind, simply say to yourself "stop." If it comes in again, say "stop" again. You'll know you've said "stop" enough times when the negative thought goes away.

Burn Those Negative Thoughts: For particularly persistent negative thoughts, write them down on a piece of paper. Get *very* negative in expressing these thoughts. Put down frustration, anger, fear, hopelessness, and pessimism about the back pain. Cuss and curse a blue streak if you wish! Then burn the piece of paper. *Don't* re-read the list; *don't* keep a copy. The idea is to release totally the negativity. If you can't burn the paper, shred it into tiny pieces and flush it.

Positive People: Hang around positive people and avoid negative people.

The Five Steps in Thought-Stopping

The following thought-stopping technique is a combination of techniques spelled out in *The Relaxation and Stress Reduction Workbook* by Davis, Eschelman & McKay, and the *Chronic Pain Control Workbook*, by Catalano. It includes some of the same elements as the techniques above and offers some variations.

1. Identification of Negative Thoughts

We have outlined this step above, as well as particular kinds of thoughts to watch for; but here are some specific examples of negative thoughts you might find: "I will never get better." "Once the pain starts, it will never stop." "It hurts so much that my life will consist of daily chronic back pain, and I don't want to live like this." "Since I have not gotten better, no doctor can cure me." "I have done exercises for three months and I cannot get better."

2. Inventory of Negative Thoughts

Now go a step further and make a *written* list of common negative thoughts and note when that thought is likely to occur. For example, at the first hint of pain, perhaps you think, "I will never get better." Note that thought down and next to it note that it came with the first sign of pain. The inventory is most important. Later you will be able to anticipate thoughts and then substitute a positive thought before the negative thought emerges.

3. Interrupt the Negative Thought

Thought stopping requires practice and training. Set an alarm or egg timer for three minutes. During this time think about a very negative thought, such as, "My back pain will never get better." When the alarm goes off or all the sand is out of the egg timer, shout "stop!" and make a demonstrable physical gesture. Stand up or snap your fingers and release the negative thought. Then think non-anxiety producing thoughts for a minimum of 30 seconds, but if the negative thought comes back again shout "stop!"

After mastering this technique, wean yourself off the alarm and shouting "stop." Then speak the word "stop" in a normal voice and once that is comfortable, whisper the word. When a whispered "stop" effectively halts the negative thought, then imagine the word "stop" being stated in the mind. Once you accomplish this, you can invoke the thought-stopping process anywhere, anytime.

4. Substitute A Positive Thought

The next phase is to substitute a positive or mind-commanding thought for the negative thought. Develop a number of alternative thoughts for each negative thought. (See the section on affirmations later in this chapter to help you write suitable substitute thoughts, or use the ones suggested below.) The substitute thoughts should be written down next to each negative thought in the negative thought inventory. The following gentle substitute thoughts are suggested by the author of the *Chronic Pain Workbook*. Breathe deeply first and affirm: "I can cope." "Relax. I can manage the pain." "The pain comes and goes." "I know how to take care of it." "The pain comes in waves. Soon it will start to abate."

For very stubborn negative thoughts, substitute "angry rebuttal statements" or "howitzer mantras" according to the *Workbook*. Often the harsher and angrier the "howitzer mantra," the more effective it can be. Curse words can also be used, if that is your style. As with the gentle substitute statement, write down the angry rebuttal or howitzer statement next to the negative thought so you will be prepared. The *Workbook* suggests these powerful thought-stopping substitute statements: "Stop this negative shit!" "Shut up with the negative stuff!" "Stop this garbage!" "No more of this helpless stuff!"

5. Journal of Negative Thoughts, Reactions and Thought-Stopping Statements and Reactions

To complete the thought-stopping process, we suggest keeping a journal to demonstrate the clear connection between negative thoughts and the body's physiological and emotional reactions. Remember, as with any technique to relieve or eliminate chronic pain, this may take time, so do not be discouraged. The journal should look like this with sample entries:

Negative Thought	Phys./Emot. Reaction	Substitution Thought	Phys./Emot. Reaction
My back hurts so much; I will never get better	muscles tighten, fear, anxiety	I can stop this pain shortly; it is only a minor flare-up, Stop this nonsense now!	muscles loosen/ calm, peace

Here are more suggestions for encouraging positive thoughts:

• Inspiring Reading: Get a book of affirmations or other inspiring reading material to read during negative times. Keep the book handy and read it on a daily basis.

• Happy Journal: Keep a "happy" journal or notebook for only positive thoughts or events. Frequently write down any healing progress no matter how insignificant it may seem as well as anything good that happens whether it's directly related to healing or to another area of life. Read and add to the "happy" book often.

• Uplifting Tapes: Listen to uplifting taped material while driving. The book, *You Can't Afford the Luxury of a Negative Thought,* is available on tape and provides nearly 12 hours of wonderful, positive listening. See your local library for other books-on-tape.

• Humor: Read Chapter 12 on the importance of humor in healing. Humor is a great way to promote optimism and positive thinking and make the shift that allows you to look at things from a new angle.

• Music: Listen to joyful music during the day. There is lots of great uplifting background music out there to listen to while you work or drive. Read Chapter 11 on music for suggestions on specific artists and titles.

• Positive Results: Focus on and talk about positive outcomes. Don't say, "I don't want to be in pain." Instead say, "I want to be strong and healthy." Being strong and healthy is the positive result, so focus on that rather than on the negative present.

Some pointers before starting and for those discouraging times:
• Be neutral: If it's too hard at first to be positive, try being neutral as an interim step. On a bad pain day, just make the observation, "I'm in a lot of pain today," without letting yourself get caught up in a cycle of negative statements like, "Oh, no! Another day like this! I can't stand it anymore! Not again! I'm so tired of hurting!" These kinds of statements only increase anguish and suffering and *don't* change the pain.
• It takes time: Remember that you may have been thinking negative thoughts for decades and it will take some time to break those old patterns of negativity. Don't expect overnight miracles. As always, be patient and gentle. Positive thinking is a *skill*—it gets easier with practice. The mental "muscles" used for positive thinking may be weak from disuse, but like physical muscles, they can get stronger with use. Exercise those "muscles" daily!
• Work on yourself: Remember that you can't change others; you can only change yourself, so change the way *you* react to your experiences and other people. While learning to be more positive, just remember to work on *yourself*, and don't worry about converting the whole world. However, two kinds of changes in others may become apparent: 1. Some will respond encouragingly, and be happy that you're more positive, (hang out with them!); 2. Others may be annoyed by your new attitude because they're of the misery-loves-company school of life (avoid them!).
• Be patient: Patience, gentleness, and compassion are the operative words for thought reprogramming. Be kind and gentle during the learning and healing process, and with those around you who may notice the growth and changes.
• Read this chapter again when discouraged.

Using Affirmations to Promote Positive Thinking
The key to changing your experience is changing your thoughts. Affirmations help you change what you *say* about the experience and changing the words can help change the thoughts. An affirmation is a short statement repeated silently or read aloud, affirming a positive outcome. It is a representation in words of positive images. Some examples might be, "I control the comfort of my body with my thoughts," or "Each day my back grows stronger and healthier."

Affirmations focus on positive outcomes (healthy, pain-free back and more functional life) rather than on a negative situation (chronic pain). Words have power. Talking about pain all the time only *keeps* the focus on the pain. Talking about, affirming, and believing in the positive desired results of pain relief and healing help bring about those results. Repeating positive affirmations on a regular basis communicates the picture of the desired result to the subconscious mind.

Writing Your Own Affirmations

Here are some tips for devising affirmations to fit specific pain-relief needs:

Short and Sweet: Make them short and easy to remember. A sentence or two at most.

Positive Rather Than Negative: Don't say "I am not in pain." or "My back doesn't ache." or "I am not tense." Rather, say, "My back grows stronger each day." or "I am relaxed."

Avoid the Future Tense: "My back will be relaxed and comfortable," makes the subconscious mind think, "Well, okay, not now, maybe later." So, use present tense statements such as, "My back is strong and healthy." Or use progressive tense statements such as, "My back is growing stronger and healthier each day."

Don't Mention It: Try not to mention what you're trying to get away from. So, as a rule, don't mention pain, discomfort, tension, or weakness in the affirmations. Use their positive opposites: ease, comfort, relaxation, strength, health, or well-being.

How and When to Use Affirmations

Repetition: This is the key. Write the affirmations on small cards that can easily be carried around. We recommend multiple sets: a pocket or purse set, some on your night stand, in the car to read at stoplights, on the bathroom mirror, or in your desk at work. The action of writing out the multiple sets is also helpful. Read them often during the day. Say them aloud whenever possible. Think them while walking or jogging.

Under Hypnosis: After reading the chapter on hypnosis, the power of affirmations with hypnosis will be clear. Once in hypnosis, repeat the chosen affirmations. If you drift off and forget the affirmations, that's okay. Just come back to the affirmations and start over.

Two Weeks: As a rule, stay with an affirmation or group of related affirmations for at least two weeks. Although there may be immediate results, keep repeating the affirmations for at least two weeks. Some affirmations may require longer to obtain results. Some affirmations may be ones to use for life, especially the ones related to positive thinking.

Keep Notes: Keep track of the affirmations, when you started, and any noticeable results.

Work on One Area at a Time: Perhaps weight loss and smoking cessation are also goals, but you cannot work on both those areas *and* pain relief at the same time. Once pain relief is achieved, use affirmations and many of the other skills in this book to make positive changes in other areas.

Patience: As always, be gentle and patient while learning this new skill. Do not get upset if a day slips by without having done affirmations. Just do them when you remember and reaffirm the desire to use this technique.

Above all, keep in mind, the most important positive belief to adhere to is your faith in the power of the program to work for you.

The Importance of Intention

Declaring your intention to be pain free and *living* that intention is another powerful, positive method to significantly reduce or eliminate pain. Keeping that intention ever-present in mind will ensure its becoming a reality. Its constant repetition will empower and motivate you to take actions consistent with this intention. For instance, with the intention always in mind, you will be more likely to remember to sit and stand properly, or to actively eliminate physical or mental stressors.

CHAPTER 5

DEEP BREATHING: RELAXATION AND PAIN RELIEF ARE A FEW BREATHS AWAY

ALTHOUGH BREATHING is something we rarely think about, it is our very connection to life. Breath work is a valuable part of any healing and pain-relief program. Proper deep abdominal breathing ensures that oxygen is distributed throughout the body. This is especially important as oxygen removes waste products from muscles in and associated with the back. Deep abdominal breathing calms the entire system and relieves anxiety. While breathing may seem to fit more logically in the section on *physical* means of pain relief, proper breathing and certain breathing techniques are necessary for many of the mental means of pain relief discussed in upcoming chapters.

What Is It?

Of course, everyone knows what breathing is. We do it day and night, awake and asleep without ceasing every single day from the moment of birth and until the last breath. It is something we probably don't think about much except when we have a cold and can't breathe easily, or when breathing is hard after exertion. Here we're talking about conscious, deliberate breathing.

The breath is a good indicator of comfort and relaxation. The breathing pattern, the speed and depth with which air is taken in, and the length of the interval between breaths, change according to both physical and emotional stimuli. However, the reverse is also true: Controlling the breath can help control the emotions. Calming the breath, calms the emotions. If you can stop and breathe, you're okay.

Why Does It Work?

Awareness of breath connects us to the present moment, the only place where pain relief can occur. It works because if you can be fully present in the moment by focusing on the breath, you think and see more clearly. When breathing is calm, so is the mind and body. Breathing and being thankful for the ever-present miracle of the breath, helps you find other things to be thankful for in the healing process and in life. Finally, proper breathing oxygenates the entire system, removing muscular waste products and promoting the healing of muscular tissue.

How Do You Do It?

Deep Abdominal Breathing:
Unfortunately, most of us do not breathe properly. In today's rushed society our breath is only inhaled to our chest and then exhaled. Proper breathing requires breathing down into the abdominal cavity and then exhaling. Follow this technique for deep abdominal breathing:
1. Sit erect on a chair with feet flat on the floor.
2. Place your hands on the belly.
3. Breathe deeply into the belly so that you feel the hands and belly rise.
4. As you exhale through the nose, feel the belly soften and contract.

Breathing Exercises for Deep Abdominal Breathing:

A variety of breathing exercises is provided here, but we suggest beginning with a simple breath-awareness exercise detailed below using deep abdominal breathing. The breath exercises are in order of difficulty, so don't jump right to *Combining Affirmations with Breathing* without first having practiced the other exercises. Always use deep abdominal breathing in all the exercises. Try all the techniques and then experiment to find out what is the *optimum time* for you to engage in a breathing technique—that is how much time you need to get relief. For example, it may take one person three minutes of breath counting to relax and feel pain reduction, but it may take five or more minutes for someone else.

Breath Awareness: Find a comfortable spot to sit or lie. If sitting, do not slump over. You want to be able to breathe in deeply and fully. If lying down, put a pillow behind the head and neck. Close the eyes. Turn the attention inward, and begin to be aware of the breath. Do not change the breathing; simply breathe normally, but pay attention. Feel the cool air coming into the nostrils and flowing down into the lungs. Feel the belly and lungs inflate. Upon exhaling, feel the air come out. Don't force the air out; just let it come out easily and naturally. Notice the pause between exhaling and inhaling. Continue to breathe and just be aware of the breath coming in and out like waves lapping upon the shore. You may notice the pause between exhaling and inhaling grows as the body calms down. Notice how the body feels. Notice if the mind wanders. If it does, just gently remind it to come back to the breath. Start with one minute of breath awareness and each day add another minute until you can spend five minutes simply breathing and being aware.

Breath Counting: The next step is breath counting to help you focus more on breath awareness. With this exercise, as above, find a comfortable, quiet spot and turn the attention to the breath. Breathe in and while exhaling, say "one." Breathe in again and when exhaling, say "two." Continue in this way up to ten and then begin again. If you lose track, start at one again. Practice this until you can to do three sets of ten counted breaths without losing track. This is an excellent way to calm and refresh the mind and body during the day.

Breathing Out Twice As Long As Breathing In: A variation of breath counting, and another good way to calm the body. Again, sitting or lying in a comfortable, quiet spot turn the attention to the breath. Focus on the breath for several breaths. Then, as you breathe in, count how long it takes to breathe in. It's not necessary to actually time the in-breath; just count. If the in-breath takes two counts, then make the out-breath last four counts. If it takes three counts to breathe in, then make the exhalation last six counts. Do this for five to ten breaths. This is an excellent exercise to do whenever you feel "spacey" or scattered during the day. It is centering and calming.

Breathing In and Out Opposite Nostrils: This type of breathing comes from Yoga. When breathing in, gently close the right nostril with the index finger so that the breath comes in through the left nostril. Then when breathing out, gently close the left nostril with the index finger so that the out breath goes out through the right nostril. Do this for 5 to 10 breaths.

Combining Affirmations With Breathing: When you can focus on the breath and stay in the moment with it, use affirmations to accompany the in and out breaths. With each pair of affirmations below, one affirmation is for the in-breath and one is for the out-breath. Think these to yourself or repeat them softly while breathing in and out. Repeat each affirmation three times (three breaths), using all seven affirmations, as an energizing, positive start to the day or as a break during the day, or choose one pair to focus on for a day or for a particular need you might have. Or create your own affirmations to use with breathing by following the guidelines for affirmations in Chapter 4.

In-breath	Out-breath
I breathe in peace and calm.	I breathe out tension and stress.
I breathe in optimism.	I breathe out negativity.
I breathe in hope.	I breathe out despair.
I breathe in energy.	I breathe out fatigue.
I breath in comfort.	I breathe out pain.
I breathe in life.	I breathe out toxins.
I breathe in gratitude.	I breathe out and smile.

Combining Imagery With Breathing: You can also combine imagery with breathing, and this combination is very powerful. Like the other breathing exercises, find a comfortable, quiet spot to do the exercises. Also, remember you don't have to see the suggested images as if watching a movie screen in order for the imagery to be effective. Here are two imagery exercises to try:

1. Find a Healing Color: If you've done the imagery exercise to find the color of the pain, then choose a healing color. Visualize breathing in this color and letting the color go to and surround the painful area. Then see the color carrying away the pain with your out-breath. Do this for several breaths several times a day.

2. Warm Sun: See yourself sitting in a favorite place in nature and feel the warm sun shining on your forehead. Breathe the sun into your body and see it going to the place that needs healing. Breathe out and see the sun carrying away the pain. Do this for several breaths several times a day.

Being in the Pause: The pause between the out-breath and the next in-breath is a wonderful place to be. It is the place where you just *are*. In relaxation exercises or self-hypnosis sessions, breathing slows as the pause between exhaling and inhaling grows. Lengthening this pause is part of what meditation is all about. People in a deep meditative state have quite long pauses between breaths. This exercise is a variation of Exercise #3 in which you breathe out twice as long as breathing in. Begin by counting the in-breath. Again if it takes two counts to breathe in, take four counts to breathe out, and then count to four before inhaling again. With the next breath, count to five before inhaling, and with the next, count to six before inhaling, if it is comfortable. See how long you can stay in the pause, but don't wait so long that you are gasping. Notice how you feel in the pause. Notice the thoughts in the pause. Notice how connected you are to the present moment. Notice how nice it is to just *be* for a few moments.

Breathing Into the Back and Other Areas of the Body: We can also direct our breath into various areas of the body that need healing. Using the instructions for breathing under breath awareness, direct the breath into the lower spine. Imagine in the mind's eye the breath moving into that area and then exhale. Use this technique to direct the breath into the lower and mid-back and flanks or any other sore area associated with the back.

Some Pointers Before You Start:

• Part of a total program: These breathing exercises are presented as part of the total program. Try them all to see which ones provide comfort and a feeling of well-being, and use those.

• Patience: Again, a reminder to be patient and gentle while practicing these techniques.

(See Appendix E for the tracks on CD #1 to be used in conjunction with this chapter.)

CHAPTER 6

BODY RELAXATION: RELAX, RELEASE, LET GO

IN THIS SECTION WE DISCUSS USING THE MIND to achieve deep physical relaxation throughout the entire body. Relaxing every muscle can be beneficial, especially if back pain is caused by muscle spasms. In terms of stress relief and overall well-being, total body relaxation is also helpful. Again this technique may seem as if it should be in the "physical means" section. However, being able to fully relax your body is essential to learning other skills in the "mental means" section.

What Is It?

Whole body relaxation is the step-by-step releasing of the major muscle groups from the top of the head to the tips of the toes. Generally this is done by first putting attention on a body part or an area of the body and tensing the muscles there, and then consciously relaxing the muscles. Tensing the muscles first helps increase awareness of the body part on which you are focusing and makes the subsequent relaxation more apparent.

Why Does It Work?

People often do not even know they are holding tension in certain areas of their bodies, or perhaps if they know, they do not quite know how to remedy the situation. Whole body relaxation puts you back in touch with the body again. The more you practice, the deeper the relaxation and the greater benefit when you learn to relax very deep muscles, especially those in the sore part of the back.

Whole body relaxation also works because when the body is deeply relaxed, you are far less likely to feel anxious. Remember that you are "bodymind," not really mind and body. Thus, as the mind can make the body tense, the loop works the other way also—if you can relax physically, you can relax mentally. *The Relaxation and Stress Reduction Workbook* tells us, "Deep muscle relaxation, when successfully mastered, can be used as an anti-anxiety pill."

71

How Do You Do It?

We suggest dictating the instructions below into a tape recorder to practice with until the whole procedure is learned by heart. We strongly recommend learning to do the procedure on your own. Being able to relax *yourself* is a very valuable and powerful tool. (We have also used an abbreviated whole body relaxation technique in the self-hypnosis sessions: the three waves of relaxation.)

Sit or lie down to do this, but if lying down, make sure the neck and head are supported. Also, do not cross the arms or legs. Let the hands rests lightly in the lap or at your sides if lying down. You will be relaxing five basic muscle groups:
• Head, face, throat, neck, shoulders, and upper back.
• Hands and arms
• Chest, abdomen
• Lower back
• Thighs, buttocks, calves, and feet.

Basically, it involves putting awareness on each area, tensing the area, and then breathing in and relaxing while exhaling. If an area remains tense after one breath, repeat until you achieve release. With each breath, say, "Breathe in relaxation; breathe out tension." Or imagery of melting may be helpful. Think or say, "Breathe in calm; breathe out and melt."

Whole Body Relaxation Procedure

1. Get comfortable: Get into a comfortable position sitting or lying. Take several deep breaths. Close your eyes.

2. Upper Body: Put attention on the scalp, and tense the muscles there. Breathe in and exhale, releasing the tension. Put attention on the face, noting any tension there, especially in the jaw. Breathe in and then exhale, relaxing and releasing the facial muscles. Note if the tongue is pushed against the top of the mouth; if it is, lower the tongue. This will relax the jaw. Let the teeth be slightly apart. Become aware of the throat, and tense the front of the neck and throat. Breathe in and release. Move around to the back of the neck, put awareness there, and tense the muscles. Breathe in and release. Move now to the shoulders and notice if you're holding them up tensely. Breathe in, shrug them up and hold them in that tense position for a second or two. Drop them as you exhale to release. Move to the upper back. Tense the muscles there. Breathe in and exhale to release. Now scan the head, face, neck, shoulders, and back. Are they relaxed? If there are still tense areas, go back and breathe into those areas and release them with the out breath.

3. *Arms and Hands:* Moving now to the hands and arms. Put awareness on the hands and all the tiny muscles and bones there. Clench your fists. Breathe in and exhale to release the fist and tension in the hands. Move to the forearms. Clenching again, breathe in and exhale to release the muscles there. Move up to the upper arms, tense those muscles as you breathe in and release the tensions with the out breath. Repeat if necessary.

4. *Chest and Abdomen:* Moving now to the chest. Become aware of that area and any tightness there. Breathe in and tense the muscles in and around the chest, and then release with the out breath. Notice that your breathing is deeper and calmer. Move to the belly. Pull the belly in with the in breath, and release it with the out breath.

5. *Lower Back:* Move attention now around to the lower back. Put awareness there and tense the muscles in and around the tailbone as you breathe in. Release with the out breath. Repeat if there is still tightness.

6. *Legs:* Moving now to the thighs. Tense the large muscles on the front of the thighs as you breathe in and relax the muscles with the exhalation. Now move to the hamstrings at the back of the thighs. Tense those muscles as you breathe in and then breathe out as you release. Now move to the buttocks, and squeeze them together as you breathe in. Relax with the out breath. Going down to the calves now, tense them as you breathe in. Release the calf muscles on the out breath. Finally, down to the feet, curl your toes in and tense all the muscles of the feet and ankles as you breathe in. Release on the out breath. Repeat for any area that remains tense.

6. *Rest:* Now simply rest for a few moments and enjoy this feeling of relaxation. Notice what it really feels like to be completely relaxed.

7. *Breathe and Stretch:* Take several deep breaths, stretch, and get up to enjoy the refreshed feeling you will experience.

(Adapted from *The Relaxation and Stress Reduction Workbook* by Davis, Eshelman, and McKay)

Learning the whole procedure should take about one to two weeks of daily practice; then you can use the abbreviated procedure outlined below:

Abbreviated Whole Body Relaxation

This is abbreviated, but it still relaxes the whole body. Use this when there isn't time to do the full body relaxation.

1. Take several deep breaths. Close your eyes.
2. Think, "Head, face, neck, shoulders, upper back," and take a deep breath, and exhale, and think, "Release." If you like the melting image, then think, "Melt" instead of "release."
3. Think, "Hands and arms," and breathe in. Exhale and think, "Release."
4. Think, "Chest and abdomen," and inhale. Breathe out and think, "Release."
5. Think, "Lower back," and inhale. Breathe out and think, "Release."
6. Think, "Thighs, calves, feet," and inhale. Exhale and think, "Release."
7. Rest for a few moments to enjoy the deep relaxation.
8. Take several deep breaths, open your eyes and smile, feeling refreshed and relaxed.

When to Use the Whole Body Relaxation
• Anxious or tense: Whenever you feel anxious or tense and there is time and opportunity to do it.
• Before sleep: Many people find it's a wonderful way to fall asleep.
• At work: Use it at work during lunch hour as a revitalizing break in the day.
• After work: Use it after work to release any tension or stress from the day and to refresh yourself for the evening.
• Before speaking to a group: If you are nervous when speaking in front of a group of people, try doing it before speaking if there's a time and place to do so. This is a good time for the abbreviated version.
• Inventory: Use it to "inventory" the body to see which parts are especially tense and the breathe into that part to relax it.

Some Pointers Before You Start
• Practice: Like other techniques in this book, whole body relaxation is a skill and you get better at it with practice. Practice daily until you have mastered all the steps. Complete physical relaxation may feel unfamiliar at first. But keep practicing until the body is trained to respond, and you will achieve deeper and more complete relaxation. So don't give up if you don't feel really relaxed the first time you try this.
• Patience: As always, patience and gentleness are the keys to teaching yourself this new skill.

CHAPTER 7

IMAGERY & VISUALIZATION: THINKING WITH THE SENSES TO RELIEVE PAIN

SIMPLY PUT, imagery is thinking not in words, but in pictures. These "pictures" may draw upon all the senses—that is seeing, feeling, hearing, smelling, or tasting an image. Visualization has a strong effect on the body because it allows direct access to the subconscious mind. For the purposes of this text, the terms imagery and visualization are used interchangeably.

What Is It?

We use visualization in everyday life. For example, imagine being at work, and your spouse calls wanting to know where something is in the garage. In the mind's eye, you picture the garage and can give that person instructions to find what he/she needs. Often when we give someone verbal directions to a place, we visualize ourselves driving or walking there and give directions based on our mind's picture. Close your eyes right now, and you can probably see your bedroom in fairly complete detail, or the house you grew up in, or any one of many familiar places. When we remember a particularly wonderful vacation or happy occasion, we often see it in our minds.

Imagery as part of a pain control program involves quieting the mind and then visualizing creative, healing, pain-relief pictures in the mind's eye. We will outline some images that have proven effective for others, but the images that you come up with will be the most powerful. Here are some examples of images that might work:

• visualizing the color of the pain as dark and dull, and changing it in the mind to a brighter, lighter, healthier color

• seeing the tight back muscles as a twisted rope, then in the mind's eye, gently untwisting the rope

• imagining golden light flowing through the sore muscles and joints

We will discuss in greater detail later how to discover the imagery that will work best for specific pain-relief needs.

Why Does It Work?

As the old adage says, "A picture is worth a thousand words," and this is certainly true when it comes to the power of imagery to change physical experience. Imagery works because it communicates most effectively with the subconscious mind. Imagination is very powerful.

We tend to think that thoughts are insubstantial because we cannot see or touch them, but they do cause real, measurable physiological changes in the body. This is because the body and mind are not really separate at all, even though for centuries Western medicine has seen them as separate entities. The mind was thought to be entirely in one's head, acting as a sort of plant operations for the factory of the body, the machinery carrying out the mind's orders. This notion is changing however. Research has shown that certain chemicals, called neurotransmitters, once thought to be manufactured and found only in the brain, can be found *all over* the body. Thus, many health-care professionals and researchers now refer to the "body-mind" to show the interconnectedness of the two. Thus, changing thoughts can change the physical experience, and one way to change thoughts is through visualization.

How Do You Do It?

You will be using the following imagery techniques: Picturing the pain-relief image in the mind's eye; as part of self-hypnosis sessions; as symbolized post-hypnotic suggestion.

Picturing the Pain-Relief Image in Your Mind's Eye

Use any one of the images below in the following way. Take three deep breaths and then focus on the selected image. For example, take three breaths, and use the twisted rope visualization previously mentioned until the pain subsides.

Pain Relief/Control Images:

• Flowing stream: Picture the pain as a flowing stream rather than as a solid object. As the stream flows by, the pain just flows away with it and disappears downstream.

• Float: Picture yourself floating above the stream with the stream being the pain, floating on by you.

• Pluck the Pain Out: Descend to a peaceful place with flowers, butterflies and birds; and smell the flowers. Pluck the pain out of the place it is in and put the pieces in a trash bag. Pull all the pieces out until you cannot feel any more pain. Close the bag covering the pieces of pain, get up, stretch, breath deeply and ascend the stair case and climb back up leaving the pain behind.

• Cool Hands: Imagine soft hands being placed over the affected area. As soon as the cool hands are placed on the body, relief is immediate.

• Warm Hands: Like cool hands, but imagine warm hands, if warmth is what you feel will relieve the pain.

• Electric Blanket: Imagine a soft, fluffy electric blanket over the affected area. Feel it grow warmer and warmer. Turn the temperature up until you get pain relief.

• Healing Green: Change the color of the pain to green, a healing color.

• Golden Light: Bathe the affected area in golden light, allowing the light to soothe and wash away pain and toxins.

• Breathe in the Sun: Imagine a favorite spot in nature, and then feel the sun on your forehead. Breathe the sunshine into the body and allow its warmth to travel to the place that needs pain relief. Allow the sunshine to stay there warming the area until relief is felt.

• Bubbles: Imagine blue and green bubbles frothing in and around the affected area, soothing, cleansing, and lightening up the pain. Then imagine the bubbles coming to the skin's surface and floating away, or popping and taking with them the pain.

• The Faucet: Imagine a faucet at the base of the spine. Open the faucet and let all the pain and tension flow out of the spine and away from the body.

• Faucet Variant: Imagine a faucet at the *top* of the spine. Turn the faucet on and let cool (or warm) water flow over the back, down off the back, taking with it the pain.

• Mountain Brook: Imagine lying by a bubbling mountain brook. Visualize lying so that your hand trails in the water. Imagine the pain coming out of the back, up the arm, out through the hand, and carried away by the stream.

• Ice Cube: Imagine the pain is an ice cube and then imagine the ice cube melting. When it has melted away, so has the pain.

• Untwist the Rope: Imagine the pain as a tightly twisted rope. Imagine the rope gently untwisting until it hangs smooth and knot-free. When the rope is smooth and unwound, the pain is gone.

•Magic Liquid: Imagine soothing, lubricating drops of magic liquid being

applied to the affected areas. Let the liquid keep dripping until the pain is gone.
• The Dimmer Switch: Imagine there is a dimmer switch in the brain. The dial goes from one to ten. One is complete ease and comfort and ten is unbearable pain. Imagine turning the dial down to one.
• The Iron Door: Focus attention on the painful area and see the nerves connected to the area as they travel up through the body to the brain where pain is registered. Imagine the pain sensations traveling up the nerves, but when they get close to the brain, a thick, iron door comes down and bars pain sensations from entering the brain and being registered.

To Use Imagery While in Hypnosis
1. Choose an image you wish to work with.
2. Follow the procedure for inducing hypnosis (the three waves of relaxation and 10-0 countdown)
3. At 0, begin working with the image, if for example, you are visualizing the pain as a twisted rope, see the rope in the mind's eye and let it unwind, "seeing" the tight muscles unwind as the rope unwinds.
4. Count up after the rope is completely unwound.

To Use an Image as a Symbolized Post-Hypnotic Suggestion
1. Choose the image. Then choose a word or phrase that *symbolizes* the desired outcome of that image. For example, with the twisted rope, the desired outcome is an untwisted rope representing smooth, tension-free back muscles. An appropriate phrase might be, "smooth rope."
2. Induce self-hypnosis.
3. At 0, work with the image, for example, with the twisted rope, follow the procedure outlined above—that is in the mind's eye, unwind the rope. But before counting back up, suggest that in waking moments, three deep breaths, and the words, "smooth rope," will make the back muscles loosen and relax.
4. Count back up.
5. You may need to work with this under hypnosis several times. Eventually, you can train the mind and body to respond in waking moments to just saying the phrase after three deep breaths, as under hypnosis.

How to Find Imagery That Works
The following section outlines how to use an image that works best for you

by finding out what the pain feels like. With a "picture" of the pain, it will be easier to choose an image. This exercise is outlined below:

1. Induce self-hypnosis.

2. At zero begin to ask the following questions and see what kind of answers come up:

• Where is the pain? Yes, in the back, but try to *see* into the place that hurts.

• What color is the pain? Dark? Light? A warm or cool color? Muddy? Dirty?

• What temperature is the pain? Hot? Cold?

• What texture is the pain? that is, what do the muscles, tendons, etc. look like in pain--twisted? frazzled? frayed? like barbed wire? hard? bumpy?

• Does the pain have a sound? sizzling, vibrating? screaming? throbbing like a drum?

• Is there a concrete object that the pain looks like? A knife stabbing into you? Flames burning you? A rat gnawing at the nerves? Needles?

Once you have some answers, tell the inner mind to remember the information. Count back up. You may not get answers to all of the above questions. For example, asking about the color, may prompt a very clear answer, "fiery red," but you may not get much from the question about how the pain sounds. These questions allow for the different ways people process information, so some questions may really spark clear answers for some people, while other questions may not call up any productive images. You may not see the pain, but rather know what it looks or feels like. That is fine.

Once you have a pain image, then either choose from the healing images we have provided or come up with one of your own. So, for example, if the pain is fiery red and feels hot, then imagery that changes the red to a cooler color, like blue or green, and of an accompanying decrease in temperature will work best. If the color of pain is muddy brown, for example, then change it to a cleaner, clearer color like green or blue, or a sunny yellow. If you can see the texture of the pain, then choose a textural image. For example, if the muscles look like a frayed and torn rope, imagine the "rope" smoothing out and all the little rips and tears healing back together. If the image is of noisy, banging pain, like a jackhammer, then imagine everything quieting down to perfect, still silence. If you visualize a specific object, then transform the object into something more pleasant: For example, transform the sharp knife into gentle massaging fingers.

Once you have a healing image that will work, then follow the instructions previously outlined for using imagery in hypnosis or in waking moments. Feel free to adapt and modify any of the above images in any way that works. Use your imagination to create other pain relief images.

Some Pointers Before You Start

It Doesn't Have to Look Like a Video: Don't get upset if you don't actually *see* an image. Seeing with the mind's eye is *not* the same as seeing with physical eyes. While many people get quite clear images, just as if watching a Technicolor movie, many people sense the image or simply know it's there. Other people may respond better to tactile imagery, that is, imagery they can feel, like a wind blowing across their skin, or the warmth of the sun on their body, or the taste of a lemon. It is *not* necessary to see photograph-quality pictures to get the benefits of imagery.

Practice: The ability to visualize *will* get better with practice. Most people can visualize and those who have trouble at first, get better at it with practice.

Any Image That Works: No matter how silly or unlikely it may seem, if it works, it is correct for you. Don't judge any images that come up while doing the receptive imagery, except to ask, "Does it work? Does it relieve my pain?" You don't have to share the images with anyone.

Trust: Trust that the image will work. It is not necessary to know how the body works to produce results. Visualize the desired result and the subconscious mind will help produce the desired outcome.

Symbol: Once you have a healing image that works, try to find a real, physical symbol for it and look at it frequently during waking moments. This could be a picture that you draw or find in a magazine. It could be a little bottle with colored water in it that represents magic liquid. It might be a seashell, a flower, or a crystal, depending on the imagery.

Patience: As always, be gentle and patient while learning this new skill.

(See Appendix E for the tracks on CD #1 to be used in conjunction with this chapter.)

CHAPTER 8

SELF-HYPNOSIS:
THE POWER OF THE SUBCONSCIOUS MIND

SELF-HYPNOSIS unlocks the door to the subconscious mind, and the subconscious mind runs the body and holds the keys to both immediate and long-term pain relief. After mastering this skill, back pain relief can be as easy as breathing deeply and saying, "No more pain." In this chapter we present a wonderful life-changing skill, and discuss how to make tapes tailored to specific pain-relief needs.

What Is It?

When many people think of hypnosis, they often imagine an intense hypnotist dangling a watch on a chain in front of a glassy-eyed subject. Self-hypnosis is relaxing the mind and body deeply to work directly with the subconscious mind to reduce, control, and relieve pain.

Hypnosis is similar to daydreaming. Have you ever stared out a window on a sunny spring day and not heard someone speak to you? Have you ever driven down the freeway in a daze and missed the exit? If so, you've experienced a light state of hypnotic trance. Hypnosis is simply an altered state of consciousness. While less aware of the immediate environment, you can actively instruct the mind because it is then more receptive. Self-hypnosis helps activate the body's natural healing intelligence.

Why Does It Work?

The subconscious mind knows how to heal the body. If you cut yourself, it knows exactly what chemicals to muster up to stop the bleeding. You do not consciously think, "Uh oh, I've cut myself. Better send some Factor H to my little toe to stop that bleeding right now!" The subconscious mind influences the body by way of the autonomic nervous system, without your *consciously* having to remind it each second, "OK, heart pump; lungs inflate; stomach digest lunch now." Self-hypnosis allows us to communicate most directly and efficiently with the subconscious mind and use its influence on the body for pain control.

How Do You Do It?

Self-hypnosis means guiding yourself by means of a simple five-step process to a place of calm and peace where the subconscious mind can be reached. Mastering the five steps of self-hypnotic induction outlined below requires time and practice, but can be done by almost anyone.

The Basic Steps in Self-Hypnosis

1. Eye fixation/breathing/eye closure: This is one of the easiest and quickest ways to enter self-hypnosis. Choose a spot just above eye level and stare at it; the spot should be just high enough to cause a bit of strain to the eyes and do not tip the chin up in order to focus on the spot. Gazing at the spot, take three deep slow breaths, in through the nose, but releasing the breath gently through the *mouth.* This method of breathing hastens physical relaxation. Go back to nasal breathing after the three breaths. Continue staring at the spot until your eyes burn a bit and you have a strong desire to close them. Upon eye closure, you will feel a nice release of tension and the pleasant relief of the closed lids over dry eyes. You have now completed the first step in the self-hypnotic induction. This step should take no more than about three minutes.

2. Three waves of relaxation: Imagine three waves of relaxation (one at a time) starting at the top of the head, flowing over the front and back of the body down to the toes, bringing deep physical relaxation to the entire body. Again this step should take only a few minutes.

3. The countdown: Counting backwards from ten down to zero, deepens the state of relaxation and brings on that special altered state of consciousness to access the subconscious. Between numbers, think or say to yourself, "going within," or "deeper, deeper," or "perfect relaxation." Zero will become, after sufficient practice, the point of perfect relaxation and calm. Practicing the ten-to-zero countdown trains the mind and body to come to complete and perfect rest at zero. Visualize walking ten steps down to a beach, or use any kind of downward imagery that works for you. For example, visualize walking down steps into a cozy basement room with an easy chair and fire, or opening ten gates down a garden path leading to a lovely garden, or floating down on a soft cloud. Use any appealing image as long as at zero you are in a peaceful, calm, safe space for you. Initially use the same image for awhile until the idea of zero as a place of perfect calm is thoroughly locked in. Later, experiment with other images. The count-down should take from three to five minutes.

4. *Make the desired suggestions:* Zero is the point where you may do affirmations, suggestions, or visualization for pain relief and healing, or simply rest at 0 and enjoy the deep, pleasant relaxation.

5. *The count-up:* After the affirmations or suggestions, count up from one to five. As with the count-down, train the mind and body to return to full awareness upon five, and on five open the eyes. Between numbers you may say, "I feel alert," or "Coming back to the here and now," or "I am alert and refreshed." The count-up is important in order not to jolt back to normal awareness; *ease* out of the hypnotic state to avoid grogginess. However, with self-hypnosis before sleep, skip the count up and simply say, "I now drift into a deep, natural sleep to wake alert and refreshed in the morning."

When and Where To Do Self-Hypnosis Sessions

Find a place and time where you won't be disturbed by phone calls, family or work demands, or loud noise. Ideally, especially while learning this new skill, practice daily. If possible, that is if your back problem allows, it's best to learn self-hypnosis sitting up in a chair with the feet flat on the floor. If you learn self-hypnosis sitting up, then you can use it almost anywhere. But if you first learn it lying down, it may be harder to enter the hypnotic state *except* when lying down. Also, some people have a tendency to fall asleep while reclining and sleep is not hypnosis. However, if sitting causes you a great deal of pain, by all means lie down on the floor, in bed, or in a recliner, whichever is most comfortable.

Making Self-Hypnosis Tapes

There are lots of excellent self-hypnosis tapes on the market covering a wide variety of subjects. But there are advantages to recording tapes:

Tailor-made Tapes: The tape can be designed for specific pain control needs and circumstances. A self-recorded tape can be more detailed and specific than a commercially-made tape for the general public ever could be. You can determine how long the pauses are, choose music, or decide if you want a tape to go to sleep with, or one to listen to in the middle of the day as a refreshing break. It's up to you.

You Know What's on the Tape: With a homemade tape, you know exactly what's on it. Generally, you cannot listen to commercial tapes before buying them and they are not often published with a script. Making tapes ensures a tape you like.

Your Own Voice: Speaking to the subconscious in your own voice, giving suggestions and affirmations you have chosen is very powerful. Being able to write suggestions and design and record scripts is a great personal growth tool.

Cost: It's cheaper! Individual commercial tapes are a minimum of $10.00 and some sets of tapes can be very expensive. You can make tapes for the price of a blank cassette.

What You Will Need to Record Tapes

A CD or tape player to play the background music (see Chapter 11 for suggestions for background music). A small hand-held tape recorder. One with a counter is helpful. A tape-script (see below).

What To Say When You Make Your Own Tapes

Refer to Chapter 3 on writing affirmations to know what to insert into the following tape-script, based on the self-hypnosis procedure outlined in this chapter. Read the script into the hand-held recorder while the selected music plays on another CD or tape player. See the information that follows about voice and rate of speech while recording. Also here is a general affirmation for back pain that can be inserted in the script if you do not want to write your own:

"The muscles in my lower (or mid, upper) back are now growing more comfortable. I feel comfort and ease flowing into this area of my back. I am doing something positive for my back now by taking these minutes to truly relax and be at peace and that peace flows into my back and through my entire body. My thoughts focus on comfort and comfort floods into my back. My mind controls my comfort level. I think comfort and then feel comfort in my back. Whenever I wish, I take three deep breaths, and think 'comfort' and my body responds, and feelings of ease and comfort flow into my back."

The Script

Introduction: The following tape-script can be used with any of the chosen affirmations or visualizations or ones suggested in this book. It is a complete self-hypnosis induction and there is an appropriately indicated space for you to insert the affirmations or imagery of your choice. Pauses are indicated by //SP// (a short pause of 1-2 seconds) or //LP// (a longer pause of 3-4 seconds).

"I am getting comfortable now. //LP// I am preparing to relax my mind and body. //SP// I choose a position that is naturally comfortable, either sitting or lying down. If I need to shift position at any time, I do, and then come back to my breath. I take a deep breath and close my eyes now. //LP// As I close my eyes I feel a sense of calm relaxation coming over my body. //SP// Now in a moment I will take three deep breaths in through my nose and release them through my mouth, gently. Ready. //SP// I take a deep breath in, and relax, release, and let go. //LP// Another deep breath in through the nose. //SP// I relax, release, and let go and exhale gently. //SP// One more deep breath in through the nose, relax, release and let go, exhaling gently through my mouth. //LP// Now breathing normally and naturally, I turn my focus within, focusing on my breath coming and going out, easily and naturally. //SP// Breathing in, I feel the air coming in and breathing out, I feel the breath leaving my body. //SP// My breath comes easily and naturally in and out. //SP//I focus now for a few moments on my breath coming and going out like waves. I know that this is time for me and for my healing. //SP// Nowhere I have to go and nothing I have to do right now except breathe, relax, release and let go....

Now I put my attention on the top of my head. //SP// With my next breath out I allow a wave of relaxation to role down over my body from the top of my head to the tips of my toes. //LP// I take a deep breath, and as I exhale, I feel a deep, soothing wave of relaxation flowing over my body. //LP// I take another deep breath and as I exhale, another wave of relaxation passes over my body as I relax, release and let go completely and sink a bit deeper into my chair or bed or sofa. //LP// One more deep breath and as I exhale a third wave of relaxation flows over my body from head to foot. //LP// I feel deeply relaxed and at ease as I continue to breathe in and out.

Now that my body is deeply relaxed, I prepare to relax my mind more deeply also. //SP// I will count from 10 down to 0, and at 0 I will be completely, profoundly relaxed in mind and body. //SP// Each number down takes me deeper into this wonderful soothing relaxed state. Each number down takes me deeper within myself to a place of peace and comfort, a place of healing and harmony. //SP// Each breath takes me deeper into the comforting relaxation. //SP//I take a deep breath now and release ... TEN //SP// deeper and deeper, more relaxed //SP// NINE //SP// deeper and deeper, more relaxed...EIGHT //SP// deeper and deeper into this lovely relaxation... SEVEN //SP// deeper and deeper down into the soothing relaxation within //LP// SIX //SP// deeper and deeper, more and more deeply relaxed and comfortable and at ease. //SP// FIVE //SP// deeper and deeper, more and more profoundly relaxed and calm //SP// FOUR //SP// calmer and calmer, more perfectly at peace //SP// THREE //SP// very calm, very relaxed now, deeper and deeper with each breath //LP// TWO //SP// very, very, calm now, calm and relaxed, calm and relaxed //LP// ONE very close now to that perfect place of peace and calm, preparing to take the final step down into deep, perfect peace and calm, each breath taking me deeper, and, //SP// ZERO //SP// perfect peace, perfect calm. I rest now and enjoy this perfect calm for a few moments. Each breath deepens the calm and peace within. A deep sense of well-being and ease fills my mind and body.

As I realize I am perfectly calm, relaxed and at ease, I will echo the following affirmations in my inner mind and these affirmations will be recorded in my inner mind, planting seeds of calm, peace, harmony, ease and healing //LP//

(Insert here the general affirmation for back comfort suggested earlier, or your own selected affirmations, which you may repeat 2 or 3 times, or insert a visualization here, then continue with the script.)

I now let these powerful healing affirmations (or images) settle deep within my inner mind, knowing that each positive word has planted a seed of peace and healing. //LP// I know that my inner mind is already at work helping me to bring these suggestions into physical reality. //SP// I know that every word has been recorded by my subconscious mind.

I know that each time I listen to this tape, I water the seeds that I have planted here today. //LP// Each time I give myself the gift of time for myself by listening to this tape, I water the seeds of greater peace and calm and healing and help those seeds to grow in my life. //LP// Each time I listen to this tape, the positive seeds I have planted here today grow stronger and more vital, crowding out the negative seeds.

I prepare now to come back to normal awareness knowing I have done something wonderful for myself today by giving myself this time for healing and these moments of deep relaxation. //LP// In a moment I will count up from 1 to 5, and on 5 I will open my eyes, feeling alert, yet calm and refreshed in both mind and body. //LP// Each number up clears my mind, and brings me closer to full awareness. I take a deep breath now and feel the energy and oxygen moving through my body. ONE //SP// feeling alert, and refreshed. TWO //SP// I take another deep breath and feel the energy surging through my body //SP// THREE //SP// More alert now, //SP// bright and alert //SP// FOUR //SP// I take another deep breath and feel the energy and vitality returning to my body as I return to full alertness and awareness of the here and how...And one more deep breath, fully aware, and FIVE //SP// I open my eyes, feeling refreshed, bright, clear-headed and alert, ready to have a wonderful day." *(This concludes the induction.)*

The Hypnotic Voice

A hypnotic voice is a bit lower and smoother than the normal speaking voice, as if talking quietly to someone in a private way, but without much inflection (ups and downs in tone). The speed is *much slower* than normal speaking speed. The first attempt at taping will probably be too fast. What seems like very slow speech when recording will probably sound too fast to your hypnotically relaxed ear, so practice first.

On the count down, from 10 to 0, speak slower and more calmly as you approach 0. Conversely, on the count up, speak with more vitality and upbeat energy as you count up to 5.

For a detailed discussion and description of the hypnotic voice and rhythm, refer to Josie Hadley's and Carol Staudacher's book, *Hypnosis For Change.*

Other Things to Consider When Making Your Own Tapes

Comfort: Be sure to sit in a position that you can comfortably maintain for the duration of recording to avoid unnecessary noise from shifting position. The noise of clothing rubbing together as you move can be picked up on the recording and be very annoying.

Don't Rustle Papers: Be careful not to flip or fiddle with the pages of the script while recording. Turn them as quietly as possible since what seems like a tiny noise while you're recording sounds much louder on the actual tape and can be very distracting.

Do Not Disturb: Find a time and place to record where you won't be interrupted by people or phone calls.

Relax: Do some deep breathing *before* recording.

Rehearse: Before taping, read your script through a few times to get familiar with it and to get used to speaking more slowly.

Volume Control: Experiment with volume of the background music. There is equipment that records voice over music, but it is expensive and unnecessary.

Pronunciation: Be careful when pronouncing words that begin and end in f, s, t, d, b, and p. If stressed, these sounds can result in distracting pops and hisses.

Try Again: Don't give up if the first tape is not all you hoped for. Blank tapes are cheap. Once you have mastered making tapes, you will have a valuable life changing tool.

There is a good source for all forms of written, audio and video hypnosis materials. Contact the following organization for a free catalog containing excellent materials:

Westwood Publishing Co., 700 S. Central Ave., Glendale, CA 91204, (818) 247-9379

(See Appendix E for the tracks on CD # 1 to be used with this chapter.)

CHAPTER 9

MEDITATION

IT'S NOT NECESSARY to go to a mountain top in Tibet to obtain or appreciate the benefits of meditation. Meditation is both simple and profound. It is simple because you just sit down, breathe, quiet the mind and focus awareness. It is profound because quieting the mind can bring about enormous changes in the way you feel and act. Meditation is highly effective in reducing pain levels and calming anxiety.

What Is It?

Just as we have experienced moments of self-hypnosis in daily life (lost in a daydream, driving past a freeway exit), we have also experienced moments of what meditation feels like: Walking along the beach, becoming one with the action of the waves; playing a game of golf or tennis, and the game just flows; everything works beautifully some days, with a feeling of being in the right place at the right time. Ram Dass, a noted meditation teacher and writer, says in *Journey Of Awakening* that these are all moments of meditation, when there is a "sense of rightness, of total perfection, of being at-one-ment, of clarity, of feeling intimately involved with everything around you." These spontaneous moments of perfection and clarity sometimes just happen, and Ram Dass tells us they "are the essence of meditation." What we want to teach in this chapter is how to actively and intentionally create more moments of clarity and perfection through meditation.

Meditation means quieting the mind by clearing it of the thought "tapes" that seem to play endlessly and then *being* in the silence. The silence is comforting in and of itself. In contrast to self-hypnosis, where the mind is quieted in order to put new ideas into it, meditation seeks to calm the thinking mind as an end in itself.

Why Does it Work?

Meditation will help with pain control and healing on a number of levels:

First, meditation provides deep relaxation, thus effectively helping those with muscle-tension-related pain. The physical changes that meditation brings about—lowered heart rate and slower breathing—have been scientifically measured, so we know meditation does cause real changes in the body. When meditating, you can reach a deep level of relaxation quickly. In fact, within minutes, meditation can bring you to the same level of relaxation that is attained *after four to six hours of sleep,* as Dr. Deepak Chopra notes in his landmark book *Quantum Healing.*

Second, the deep relaxation of meditation improves general health and well-being. Long-term meditators have been shown to decrease their biological age by five to twelve years. A Blue Cross/Blue Shield study cited in *Quantum Healing* looked at 2000 meditators in the mid-1980s, and found the group much healthier, both mentally and physically, than the American population in general. The meditators were hospitalized 87 per cent less often for heart disease and 50 percent less often for tumors than the non-meditators in the study.

Third, meditating helps you deal with adversity in a calmer, balanced way. At first this state will be experienced only during meditation. But continued regular meditation will help you access calmness when not meditating, to operate from a place of calm within. This benefit of meditation is less tangible than the first two, and the changes will be subtle, but cumulative.

Fourth, meditation helps you be more aware of the thoughts and feelings you have about pain. We have talked at length about how thoughts and feelings influence, indeed even create, our experience, so it is useful to see what exactly our thoughts and feelings are. When meditating, you discover an objective distance from thoughts so as to observe them, rather than be entangled in them. Think of the mind as a pond and each thought as a pebble dropped into the pond. Many pebbles dropped into the pond agitate and muddy the waters. In order to see clearly, the pond must be still. That is what meditation does.

Finally, meditation connects you with a higher spiritual source. We will talk in more detail about faith and prayer in a later chapter, but whether you call it God, a Higher Power, or the Universe, connecting with this source can be very beneficial.

How Do You Do It?

People have meditated for centuries all over the world. There are many different ways to meditate and many books written on it. To find out more about meditation, how to do it, and perhaps about meditation retreat centers, we recommend *Journey of Awakening* by Ram Dass. A trip to the local public library or bookstore will provide access to the many books on meditation.

In this chapter we will present a very simple way of meditating. If you have tried the breathing exercises, these are the first steps in the meditation process. If you have not read the chapter on breathing and not tried the breathing exercises, go back and do that before going on.

Where to Meditate

As with the self-hypnosis sessions, choose an appropriate place where you won't be disturbed. Choose a comfortable chair with a back for support and place feet flat on the floor. Don't slump over because it will block full breathing. It is preferable to sit rather than lie down to avoid falling asleep. We have also provided instructions here for a walking meditation that can be done indoors or out depending on the weather. Be sure the walking area is safe and obstacle free to avoid tripping or falling

How to Meditate

There are many ways to meditate and many different practices the world over. We offer three simple variants here.

Simple Sitting Meditation:

1. Sit in the chair, back straight, but not stiff, feet flat on the floor, hands loosely lying in your lap, not clasped. Close your eyes.

2. Take a few slow, deep breaths.

3. Begin to focus on the breath, just noticing how it feels coming in and going out. Do not change the breath; simply notice it.

4. Focusing more on the breath, say quietly to yourself, "I am breathing in" on the in-breath, and "I am breathing out" on the exhale. Do this for several breaths.

5. Now as you breathe in and out, notice the pause after the out-breath before the next in-breath. Just notice that pause for several breaths. Notice if the pause gets longer as you relax.

6. Now in the pause, think to yourself, a calming phrase like, "Going within," or "Peace and calm." Continue to do this, breathing in easily and naturally, thinking the phrase in each pause. If the mind wanders just come back to the breath and the calming phrase.

7. Initially, start with five minutes a day. (It doesn't sound like much, but for

many people *really* stopping for just five minutes is difficult.) When you can sit for five minutes, and stay centered on the breath, go to ten minutes. Build up to twenty minutes.

Flower Meditation:

1. Choose a fresh flower—any type will do, though one that is fragrant would be best.

2. Sit comfortably, feet flat on the floor, and hold the flower gently in your hands in the lap.

3. While looking at the flower, take three deep, slow breaths, in through the nose and release them gently through the mouth. Continue gazing at the flower and take several more breaths, calming the mind and body as you focus on the breath.

4. Now bring the flower slowly up to the nose and breathe in its scent. Take several more deep, slow breaths while smelling the flower. Return the flower to your lap and close the eyes.

5. Now with eyes closed, bring the flower up to your cheek and gently brush it with the flower petals. Feel their smoothness.

6. Now simply picture in the mind the flower. Picture its perfection, its freshness.

7. Now in your mind, gently echo this affirmation three times: "I am as naturally perfect as this flower."

8. Silently give thanks for the beauty of this flower, and all flowers, and for the perfection that flowers represent. Take a deep breath, smile, and open your eyes.

Walking Meditation:

This can be done indoors or out, weather permitting. If sitting still is hard for you, try this meditation. If indoors, make sure there is enough space to walk 6 to 8 paces before turning. The point of walking meditation is to tune into your own body, breathing, and natural pace, and to become more aware of the body and how it moves.

1. Begin by standing straight and tall, but not stiff.

2. In place take three deep breaths, in through the nose and release gently through the mouth. Keep the eyes open.

3. Focus awareness on the breath for a few breaths.

4. Now breathe out, and on the next in-breath, step forward on the right foot. Place the right foot firmly on the ground and balance yourself, but begin to just roll the left foot off the floor.

5. Breathe out and gently, mindfully, lift the left foot, stepping forward onto it

as you exhale. Begin to roll the right foot off the floor as you prepare to inhale again.

6. Bringing the right foot up and forward, inhale fully and place the right foot down.

7. Continue in this way: breathing in when stepping with the right foot, and out with the left foot. If indoors, continue for a total of 8 steps and then turn around. If outdoors, be aware of the connection to the earth.

This slow pace may be hard at first, but with practice, you will find this meditation very refreshing.

When to Meditate

Especially when first learning to meditate, daily practice is best, and once the benefits are evident, you will probably want to continue the daily practice. Anytime is a good time to meditate, but there are pros and cons to the various times. Try different times to see which works best. Choose a time when you won't be disturbed and when you won't fall asleep. Also, most meditation books recommend not meditating right after a meal; you may fall asleep. However, if you are hungry, a growling stomach may be distracting.

Morning: Many people find meditation a wonderful way to start their day, and feel scattered and frazzled all day if they miss their morning meditation. Nothing seems to go right. If you're a "morning" person, morning meditation may be nice. However, some people may feel too sleepy in the morning and fall asleep when they try to meditate.

Lunch-time: If this is an option at work or school, that is if you have a quiet, private place, a lunch hour meditation is a great way to refresh yourself in the middle of the day.

Afternoon: Meditation in the late afternoon can be refreshing and will help clear the late afternoon mental "fog" that sometimes strikes at about 4:00.

After work: Meditating when you come home from work is an excellent way to release the stress of the workday and refresh yourself so you can enjoy the rest of the evening with family or friends.

Before sleeping: Meditating before bed helps release concerns and tension so that you can sleep peacefully. However, when first learning to meditate, you may fall asleep, so bedtime may not be the best time to *learn* to meditate, but later it can be a wonderful way to relax into sleep.

Some Pointers Before You Start

Distracting thoughts: If troubled by these while meditating, that's normal. Try to visualize them as clouds and let them blow away. If they come back, do not get distressed. If they are persistent, just keep breathing and focusing on the breath until the thoughts calm down.

Write it down: If you suddenly remember something you must do and can't let go of the thought or are afraid you may forget, then write it down on a pad next to you and return to meditation. Once the thought is on paper, let it just pass through the mind when it comes up, without worrying you'll forget it.

Explore: We have presented a basic meditation technique. You may wish to explore meditation in more depth. Volumes have been written on the subject and we can't possibly describe all the different techniques and uses of meditation. Check out the many books on the subject and numerous meditation groups all over the country if you wish to delve more deeply. Also, there are many audio and video tapes available on this subject.

Simple, but not easy: While the practice of meditation is simple, it's not easy. Be patient and gentle while learning this technique. Your meditation practice may have the same highs and lows of everyday life. Some days it will be easy; other days it will be harder to calm the mind. Just remember the day it's the hardest is probably the day you most need to do it!

(See Appendix E for the track on CD # 1 to be used with this chapter.)

CHAPTER 10

OUT OF PAIN ISOLATION: CONNECTING WITH OTHERS

CHRONIC PAIN DEBILITATES AND ISOLATES. After being in pain for an extended period of time, you may begin to withdraw both physically and emotionally from family members, friends, and co-workers because it is hard to be cheerful when in pain, and it requires effort to smile and carry on the normal social interaction that grows and sustains relationships.

Perhaps family, friends, and work mates were attentive and supportive in the early stages. But after many weeks or months, that initial burst of support may have faded. You are not only in pain, but alone and lonely as well. This chapter is designed to help relieve this loneliness and isolation.

What Is It?
Connecting with others means initiating and nurturing new, or rekindling lapsed, relationships with the people around you, from family members to the community. This can be as simple as a phone call to a friend or as involved as joining a weekly support group or doing community volunteer work.

Why Does It Work?
When you are in pain, it is natural to turn inward as you struggle to cope. However, it can lead to becoming obsessive and too self-involved. There is a danger that the pain and the body's response to it will become your primary focus and entire reality. Connecting with others shifts attention away from yourself, and also helps keep you busy and distracted from pain.

The isolation of chronic pain increases suffering, and this in turn leads to more isolation. Thus, coming out of the shell of isolation is important to the healing process.

Connecting with others creates a positive feedback loop. At first, it may take some effort to initiate and maintain new relationships or rekindle old ones. But you will find that connecting will make you feel better, and when you feel better, it will be easier to build and maintain relationships.

How Do You Do It?

There are many ways to connect. Social activities with friends, outings and romance with your significant other, and activities and time with your children should be planned for and monitored on the weekly charts.

We are not, of course, suggesting you must do *all* these things. Choose those activities that are appealing, and revise or adapt according to your lifestyle, time, and energy. It is hoped that looking at the list might spark interest in connecting again and offer ideas about how to connect. The only proviso is that you relate in a positive way to positive people.

We have set up the following suggestions, starting with family, moving out to friends, to work, and out to the larger world of the community. Start wherever you like. Start small, with family and friends, and then move out to the community when you're ready.

Ways to Connect with Family

• Rent videos and pop popcorn on a Friday or Saturday night.
• Have a family "slumber party"—rent videos, get pizza, camp out in sleeping bags together in the family room; kids get to stay up as long as they can keep their eyes open (not on a school night!).
• Take walks, go for bike rides, or walk the dog together.
• Plan, shop for, and cook a special meal together.
• Plant a window, patio, or backyard herb garden and nurture the garden together.
• Make one night a week "special" when everyone is all home together and has a meal together.
• Look at old family photo albums together, or make a project of gathering and organizing family photos.
• Make one night a week "joke" night when everyone has to come to the dinner table with a joke or funny story to share.
• Have "secret pal" week when family members leave little notes or small gifts for other family members.
• One night a week, have everyone come to the family dinner table with a positive

statement for each family member—such as, "Mom, I appreciate your hard work."
• Put special notes in loved ones' lunch bags that say, "I love you."
• Plan a family reunion with extended family.
• Bring home flowers for your partner for no reason.
• Write notes or cards to family members you haven't seen in years.

Ways to Reconnect With Friends

• Be sure to talk to at least one friend, outside of work, every day, either in person or by phone.
• Share jokes with friends in person, by phone, fax, or e-mail.
• Write notes to old friends you haven't seen in years and reconnect.
• Invite friends over for "film festivals" of favorite old films on video.
• Go to your next high school or college reunion.
• Do a " progressive" dinner: appetizers at one house, main course at another, and dessert at yet another.
• Bake cookies and take them to a friend.
• Give a party.

Ways to Connect with People at Work

• Each day be sure to say something positive to someone, whether it's a compliment on a new hairstyle, or praise for a job well done.
• Start a brown bag lunch-time book discussion club.
• Start a potluck lunch club—perhaps on Fridays, everyone signs up to bring something to share.
• Start a lunch-time meditation group.
• Start a lunch-time positive thinking discussion group.
• Have lunch at least once a week with someone just for companionship, rather than business.
• Have brown bag picnics with work mates in nice weather if your work site environment permits.
• Bring in homemade cookies once in awhile for everyone.
• Find out when people's birthdays are, get a card, and take it around for everyone to sign.

Ways to Make New Connections

• Join a book discussion club, or start one in your area.

• Start a Neighborhood Watch group if there isn't one in the neighborhood.

• Bake cookies and take them to a neighbor you haven't met.

• Take classes. Check out the local recreation department for classes in arts and crafts, exercise, and photography. Check out the adult school or community college for classes available in a wide variety of subjects.

• Join a fitness center.

• Go on a cruise or organized tour with a group.

• Join a local little theater group.

• Join a special interest group such as the Sierra Club.

• If you're single, check out local singles' groups in the area.

• If you're a single parent, look into Parents Without Partners.

• Join a local meditation group.

• Get on-line with a computer network and connect with people all over the world who may share common interests with you.

• Join a support group.

• Make an effort to create small positive connections when shopping and taking care of the day-to-day business of life. Smile and make a cheerful comment to grocery clerks, bank tellers, the mail carrier, or the garage mechanic. Remember that when you put out positive, cheerful energy, that's what you attract.

Reaching Out to the Community

Volunteer work in the community is an excellent way to feel better and to venture out of the isolation of chronic pain. It is a way to make new connections in a positive, loving way. Each of us has unique abilities that can be a gift to others, and it is very rewarding and healing to share these gifts.

It is possible you are already aware of volunteering opportunities in the community, but we offer some suggestions here to get started if you do not know how or where to get connected to volunteer. The suggestions are in two categories:

• suggestions for people and places that often need volunteers

• specific organizations that need volunteers.

People and Places Around You as Sources of Volunteer Work

Church or synagogue: Your church or synagogue may sponsor programs in the community.

Schools: If your children are in school, schools often need volunteers for a variety of activities from the PTA to fundraising to library workers.

Youth sports leagues: Little League baseball and AYSO soccer need coaches.

Political campaigns: These are largely run with volunteer help and require phone answerers/canvassers, envelope stuffers, etc.

Public broadcasting: The local public radio or television station probably runs pledge drives and this is often done with volunteer help.

Hospitals: Volunteers fill a variety of duties at hospitals.

Food banks: Find out if the community has a local food bank. Food banks need food, but they also need people to inventory, organize, and stock food supplies as well as deliver and pick up food.

Libraries: Check with the local library to see if they have a literacy program in which you could be a volunteer reading tutor, or if they have a program in which volunteers read to the blind.

Specific Organizations That Need Volunteers

Check the phone book for local listings of the following organizations:

Meals On Wheels: They need people to deliver hot, cooked meals to elderly or ill individuals in their homes.

Big Brother or Big Sister: They match up individuals with underprivileged children to give these children a positive adult role model.

Catholic Charities: They run a variety of programs, all over the US and the world. They need volunteer clerical help, and volunteers for their grocery-buying and meal-delivery services for the ill or elderly.

Jewish Community Federation: They have an extensive, nationwide Volunteer Placement Program with a wide variety of services and programs.

Mission Hospice Inc.: The Hospice organization trains volunteers to care for terminally ill and dying patients in their homes, and to support the families of these patients by providing respite care. There will be training required in order to work for this organization.

Some Pointers Before You Start

Avoid burnout: Remember, reconnecting with and helping others is just a part of a whole healing program. Working with the program outlined in this book does require a time commitment, so pay attention to your own mental and physical energy levels. Take it a step at a time, one day at a time. Don't overextend.

Your talents: Consider what your unique talents are and how you could use them to help others, whether it's family, friends, co-workers, or the community.

Do your homework: Find out exactly what you are committing to in terms of time, training, and tasks involved.

Do something you love: Do volunteer work that speaks to your heart and for which you have a strong personal interest and commitment.

CHAPTER 11

MUSIC AND SOUND: HARMONIC JOURNEY TO PAIN RELIEF

What Is It?

MUSIC IS PART OF OUR EVERYDAY LIVES. We listen to it in the car, at home, at work, in elevators, and while shopping at the mall. Music is a powerful emotion-altering medium. It can sadden or elate, excite or depress; it can make us melancholy, anxious or fearful. Music's great power to soothe anxiety and relieve pain is a wonderful tool in a pain management program.

Why Does It Work?

Music can relieve pain because it affects our emotions. Each of us reacts differently to various types of music. In *Healing Music* by Watson and Drury, the authors quote a study by Kate Hevner, who classifies music into eight categories in terms of the listener's mood response: These include: 1. solemn and sacred; 2. sad and doleful; 3. tender and sentimental; 4. quiet and soothing; 5. sprightly and playful; 6. joyous and happy; 7. exhilarating and exciting; and 8. vigorous and majestic.

The authors also refer to Nevill Drury's framework for music which categorizes music based on the five elements central to a number of "metaphysical systems, including yoga, astrology, tarot and western alchemical mysticism." These elements are: "Earth (level of everyday consciousness), Water, Fire, Air, Spirit (transcendental awareness)."

Music changes our moods instantly. Just think how scared you may have been in the movie *Jurassic Park* when the music heralded the approach of the T. Rex, or how patriotic when hearing "The Star Spangled Banner" at the opening of sporting events, or how relaxed when listening to soothing harp music. Music therapy is used daily throughout the country to help the mentally ill, in orthodontist offices to calm the fear of pain, and in cardiac units in hospitals to relax patients recovering from open heart surgery. Music distracts us from pain, calms our anxiety, and focuses us away from pain. Music "quiets the mind" according to Watson and Drury. Music can even, through chanting, prepare individuals to walk through burning coals or allow Native Americans to achieve a trance-like state so they can participate in traumatic and painful initiation rituals. According to *Healing Music*, music's great power is that it focuses the mind, and with a focused mind, virtually anything can be accomplished.

How Do You Do It?

It's simple; just listen to music. We recommend music to change mood when necessary, but at a minimum of at least 30 minutes a day. Soothing music as an environmental background at work or at home is even better. The key is to find the right music to bring on the right mood. There is certain music to avoid because it may prompt a negative mood response. Sad and doleful, maudlin, or any type of music or particular song that reminds you of a sad or disturbing time, or evokes negative emotions is *not* suitable. To make it easy to find music to suit your mood and purpose, we have classified some music below:

Quiet, Soothing Music: Ideal For Meditation or Relaxation

Crystal Suite	Steven Halpern
Dreamflight	Herb Ernst
Gate of Sanctuary	David & Steve Gordon
Lost Oceans	John Huling
You Are the Ocean	Gilead Limor
Interludes: Timeless Sea	Steven Gruskin

Happy and Playful Music: To Elevate Your Mood

Rain Dance	Phillip Elcano
After the Rain	Rod Brown
Island	Chris Glassfield
Freefall	Malcolm Harrison

Exhilarating and Exciting: To Pump You Up

I'm So Excited	Pointer Sisters

Seriously Live	Phil Collins
Thriller	Michael Jackson
Once Upon a Time	Donna Summer
Flashdance	Movie Soundtrack

Vigorous and Majestic: To Inspire You

Jurassic Park	Movie Soundtrack
Silverado	Movie Soundtrack
Superman	Movie Soundtrack
Star Wars	Movie Soundtrack
Braveheart	Movie Soundtrack
Last of the Mohicans	Movie Soundtrack

This is, of course, only a sampling. We suggest consulting the book *Healing Music* for a more exhaustive list, or contact the following New Age music companies for a catalog:

> Environments by Syntonic Research, Inc.
> (environmental sound tapes)
> 3405 Barranca Circle
> Austin, TX 78731-5711   (512) 459-4345
>
> Inner Peace Music by Mary Richards
> (music for relaxation and meditation)
> 881 Hawthorne Drive
> Walnut Creek, CA 94596 (510) 945-0941

Obviously, this is only a partial listing of the vast array of music available, but it will get you started. Many concerts, performances, and music videos also now appear on video tape. Video tape enhances the effect of music through the visual stimulus. We suggest visiting a local CD/tape store, large bookstores, and also the public library to explore the musical possibilities to enhance the pain management program.

CHAPTER 12

HUMOR AND LAUGHTER: POWERFUL PAINKILLERS

HUMOR AND LAUGHTER are amongst the most powerful pain relievers. Throughout our lives we have experienced and enjoyed humor and laughter. Indeed, the old saw, "Laughter is the best medicine" may be trite, but its truth has been proven over and over again. In *Anatomy of an Illness*, Norman Cousins reported "that ten minutes of genuine belly laughter had an anesthetic effect and would give [him] at least two hours of pain-free sleep." Cousins cured himself of collagen disease, a serious and painful disorder of the connective tissue, through a combination of large doses of Vitamin C and a steady diet of comedy, including The Marx Brothers, Three Stooges, and Candid Camera. In *The Healing Power of Humor*, Allen Klein commented upon Cousins' experience: "Cousins knew about the connection between unmanaged stress and illness. He reasoned that if negative emotional states played a part in his disease, then perhaps positive emotions could help him get well." Humor and laughter help foster positive emotions.

Why Do They Work?

Humor and laughter are of tremendous value in healing and relieving pain because they have both physiological and psychological benefits:

Physiological Benefits: Laughter has the power to stimulate the production of endorphins. Klein explains that laughter has definite effects both inside and outside the body, and when "we are engaged in a good, hearty laugh, every system in our body gets a workout." On the outside, he says, "you may have bounced up and down, rocked back and forth, or doubled over from time to time. Your mouth was probably wide open in an effort to take in more air. Tears may have been streaming down your face." However, on the inside, "mirthful laughter affects most, if not all, of the major physiologic systems of the human body. Your cardiovascular system…was being exercised as your

105

heart rate and blood pressure rose and then fell again. Your heavy breathing created a vigorous air exchange in your lungs and a healthy workout for your respiratory system. Your muscles released tension as they tightened up and then relaxed again. Finally, opiates (endorphins) may be released into your blood system, creating the same feelings that long distance joggers experience as 'runner's high.'" Twenty seconds of laughter, according to Klein, gives the heart the same workout as three minutes of heavy rowing!

Psychological Benefits: Klein also explains that humor gives us four critical psychological benefits: 1. power; 2. the ability to cope; 3. the proper perspective; and 4. balance. The importance of each of these for the chronic pain sufferer is clear. Concerning power, Klein explains, "In laughter, we transcend our predicaments. We are lifted above our feelings of fear, discouragement, and despair. People who can laugh no longer feel sorry for themselves" but rather, "feel uplifted, encouraged and empowered." Klein notes that humor helps us cope because it "draws our attention away from our upsets...can diffuse stressful events...(and) acts to relieve fear." Humor relieves tension surrounding serious events, helps create a positive attitude, and allows us to stop worrying and get on with our lives. Regarding perspective, Klein asserts that humor allows us to step back and see "ourselves and upsets in a new way ... and taking a humorous approach reveals new insights and possible solutions to our problems." Merriment helps us keep a healthy balance because, as Klein states, humor gives us "a way out" before we reach states of depression or suicide. According to Klein, chronic pain can cause people to "take themselves and the world so seriously and get so caught up in their dilemmas that they cannot see any way out. When individuals find comedy in chaos, they are no longer caught up in it, and problems become less of a burden."

How Do You Do It?

Humor is such a powerful pain reliever we recommend devoting time each day to the humor requirements of our program. Follow these important steps and tickle the funnybone with hilarity from the source list below:

• View, listen to, or read humor for $^1/_2$ hour from the humor source list.

• Spend 15 minutes a day telling your family, friends or work associates two funny jokes discovered while viewing, listening to, or reading humor.

• Write down in a loose-leaf notebook those jokes to build a library of jokes.

The Humor Source List

Humor can be found almost anywhere, any time, day or night. We guarantee great laughs, the potential release of endorphins, and achievement of many of the physiological and psychological benefits noted above. Simply put, laughter is the best medicine. Check these sources out:

• Television offers a great variety of humor programs. TV sitcoms offer lots of laughs. Watch or record any of the following: *Cheers, I Love Lucy, Jerry Seinfeld, Friends, Frazier, Mad About You,* or *Saturday Night Live.* Record on VCR some of those listed or at least audio tape the sound tracks for future reference. Sitcoms contain many of the best belly laughs. Standup Comedy is offered on the Comedy channel, VH1, MTV, Lifetime Television and other cable networks, as well as local stations. David Letterman and Jay Leno offer terrific jokes and funny commentary on current events in their nightly monologues. The best bet is to audio tape the monologues and then listen again to select your favorite jokes. Cable TV offers great comedy movies and comedy concerts. View them, and video tape favorites so you can review them when down or discouraged.

• Audio and Video Sources: The library or video store has large collections of comedy tapes to borrow or rent. Check movie listings and read reviews to find movies that are rated high in humor. A few suggested comedians, who provide some of the best belly laughs: Three Stooges, Billy Crystal, Jay Leno, Marx Brothers, Eddie Murphy, David Letterman, Rosie O'Donnell, Bill Cosby, Woody Allen, George Burns, W.C. Fields, Laurel and Hardy, Jonathan Winters, Rodney Dangerfield, Robin Williams, Whoopi Goldberg, and Roseanne Barr.

• Books: At the library you'll find anthologies of humor, great joke books, cartoon books, parodies, satire, compendiums of puns, riddles, humorous quotes, treasuries of anecdotes, and comedy celebrities' wit and wisdom. Look for the comedians noted above, and/or check out books by some of the following: Woody Allen, Erma Bombeck, Art Buchwald, Gary Larson, Leo Rosten, Gary Trudeau or the Calvin & Hobbes cartoons. Used book stores, swap meets, flea markets, and garage sales are other sources for inexpensive humor books.

• Computer Sources: A computer with a modem makes the world of humor a mouse-click away. In each of the commercial on-line services including Compuserve, Prodigy, America On-Line, and Delphi, there are sections on humor from which you can download thousands of jokes. On the Internet there are numerous sections, forums, usenet groups and World Wide Web pages that contain archives of humor. To find humor on the World Wide Web, type laughter and humor on your favorite search engine. Humor pages will be listed. The Internet probably has the best and most current collection around. Refer to *The Internet Yellow Pages* by Hahn and Stout for a full listing of humor resources on the Internet. If your computer has CD-Rom capability, you really are in luck. Each CD-Rom can store an encyclopedia's worth of information. The following listed CD-Roms contain in total over 500,000 categorized jokes to print out. They include: *A Million Laughs*, by Interactive Publishing; *Speech Clips Library* by Aces Research; *The Complete Bookshop*, by Chestnut CD-Rom; *Insane Impersonations*, by Chestnut CD-Rom; *Speakers Encyclopedia*, by Interactive Media Pursuits; and *Jokes & Pranks*, by Racecar Publishing.

• Newspapers and Magazines are a plentiful source for humor through cartoons, comics and columns. Generally, there is at least one humorous columnist in the newspaper, and often, papers have humorous filler pieces throughout. Nearly all magazines from *Reader's Digest* to *Playboy* to the *New Yorker* have cartoons. Cut those out that really make you laugh and keep them in a notebook or folder to peruse for a quick "dose" of humor medicine.

• Family, Friends and Work Associates: Under our humor plan, you will have to tell at least two good jokes a day. Friends, family, and co-workers are the best sources of current humor. Why not get a joke in return from those you tell jokes to? There are many people in different job capacities who need humor to promote their business or profession. Try a couple of these folks for good jokes: doctors, dentists, real estate agents, stockbrokers, salesman, car mechanics, book store owners, waiters and waitresses, ministers, priests or rabbis, and neighbors. If you are lucky enough to know some really funny and positive people, spend more time with them.

Bonus Humor Exercises: While not required in the program, try a few of these humor exercises or techniques for additional hours of pain relief.

• Take classes at a local community college on humor, how to tell jokes, or on the history and science of humor and laughter.

• Learn to imitate funny comedians.

• Contact local hospitals to see if they have a humor therapy program you can enroll in or at least obtain a copy of their reading, audio and video cassette lists. The Duke University Comprehensive Cancer Center, in Durham, North Carolina contains one of the most extensive lists of humor in America used in treating cancer patients. Write them for a copy.

• Play various comedy games including Charades, The Improv Comedy Game, Pictionary, and other commercial or non-commercial games that have a comedy theme to them.

• Read these books for many more humor and laughter techniques: *The Healing Power of Humor,* by Allen Klein; *Laugh After Laugh,* by Raymond Moody; *Humor as Therapy,* by Thomas Kulman; and *The Laughter Prescription,* by Laurence J. Peter and Bill Dana.

No doubt we've left off a favorite comedian, book, or movie, but our abbreviated list will at least get you started. Remember, you must laugh and pick out some jokes for retelling to others. You really can't beat this form of pain relief.

(See Appendix E for the track on CD # 1 to be used with this chapter.)

CHAPTER 13

FAITH AND PRAYER:
THEIR PLACE IN A PAIN MANAGEMENT PROGRAM

FAITH AND PRAYER can play a valuable role in a pain management program. Whatever faith you ascribe to, prayer practice can strengthen and enhance the pain management program. However, you will get better results with faith and prayer if they are an everyday part of life, not just once a week in church or temple. Those with more agnostic leanings can still pray. Even those who do not believe there is a supreme being called God can pray and have faith—in the healing process.

What Is It?

The dictionary defines faith as "a confident belief in the truth, value, or trustworthiness of a person, idea, or thing." Thus, we are not asking you to believe in God if you don't, but rather to believe that the body has a natural healing intelligence, and that there is order and creative intelligence in the universe, whether it is called God, Jehovah, Allah, Goddess, the Tao, the Almighty, Infinite Intelligence, or the Healing Principle Within. This intelligence and order is always at work for the highest good of all beings, even though it may not always appear that way. The dictionary further defines faith as "belief that does not rest on logical proof or material evidence." That fits perfectly with what we've been saying about the mind and pain relief. Years of medical training are not necessary to use the mind to heal the body. You don't have to know consciously or logically how a bone knits itself back together when it's broken. The body knows how to do this because of its own natural intelligence, a reflection of the natural intelligence at work in the universe.

Prayer is a natural outgrowth of faith, and is simply the act of speaking to this creative intelligence and putting yourself in alignment with the natural order of the universe. Prayer is affirming confidence in this creative intelligence and in the body's ability to get better.

Why Does it Work?

Scientists have been looking at why and how prayer works for over a century. The results of studies testing the effects of prayer on medical patients showed without a doubt that prayer works. In his book *Healing Words*, Dr. Larry Dossey tells us, "Experiments with people showed that prayer positively affected high blood pressure, wounds, heart attacks and anxiety." Dossey was so impressed with the data that he decided that "not to employ prayer with [his] patients was the equivalent of deliberately withholding a potent drug or surgical procedure." The experiments also showed that it did not matter if the praying person was in the presence of the person being prayed for or at some distance. Prayer still worked. It was even able to penetrate lead-lined chambers and still affect the prayed-for subject. As Dossey says, "Nothing seemed capable of stopping or blocking prayer."

Although many scientists remain skeptical about prayer, there is still reason to pray. Even if the mechanism by which prayer effects healing cannot be scientifically pinned down, prayer is valuable for its own sake. In the nineteenth century, Sir Francis Galton, an English scientist, cited in Dossey's book, said of prayer: "A confident sense of communion with God must necessarily rejoice and strengthen the heart and divert it from petty cares...[and those who pray] can dwell on the undoubted fact that there exists a solidarity between themselves and what surrounds them...that they are descended from an endless past, that they have a brotherhood with all that is, and prayer can bring serenity during the trials of life."

Thus, whether you believe in God or not, prayer brings serenity and makes you feel better emotionally, spiritually and physically.

How Do You Do It?

Prayer will work best if it is part of everyday life, and so this section will suggest ways to incorporate prayer into daily life. If you already have a prayer practice, this chapter may offer some new ideas to enhance it. If you've never prayed or have not prayed since childhood, this chapter offers some practical advice about how to begin praying and shows just how simple prayer really is.

We use the word God below in the instructions, but please note that anywhere the word God is used, you may substitute any name for him/her/it which makes you comfortable and expresses your understanding of God or the universe. Here are some suggestions: Higher Power, the Absolute, Mother-Father God, Infinite Intelligence, the Universe, the Almighty, the Tao, the Healing Principle Within, the Christ Within, Living Loving Presence, One Power/One Presence, Life Force, the Light, Prime Cause, I Am, All That Is, or any other name that works for you. If you are agnostic or are uncomfortable with using the name God, simply pray to the natural healing intelligence within the body.

When to Pray

Morning: Upon waking, prayer is a good way to set a positive tone for the day.

At night: Before sleeping, prayer is a good way to encourage healing and tranquillity while sleeping.

In the shower: Allow the water to flow over you for a moment and use that moment to pray.

Anytime: When you feel the need to be centered, calmed, uplifted, or encouraged, take a few deep breaths, and pray silently wherever and whenever you need to. Even 30 seconds of prayers can be beneficial.

Progress: When you see or feel some pain relief progress, take a moment to acknowledge the progress and give a little prayer of thanks.

Before or during meditation: Take a moment before meditation to pray to get into a tranquil, prayerful mode, and to dedicate the time to healing, and/or while meditating, use a short prayer as a centering device.

What to Say When You Pray

In her book, *Your Body Believes Every Word You Say*, Barbara Hoberman Levine, says of prayer, "If you think you don't know how to pray, relax! It's just like talking to someone you love and trust, in your own words, in silence, or aloud, wherever you happen to be--sitting, standing, walking, lying down or even driving." Prayer does not require "thee" and "thou" to work. Simple, clear language from the heart works. The guidelines for prayer are similar to those for writing affirmations; in fact, affirmations are really a kind of prayer. You can change affirmations into prayers easily. Review the section on how to write affirmations in Chapter 4 and then change the affirmations into prayers by acknowledging the presence and working of a divine intelligence. Some examples of affirmations turned into prayers might be:

Affirmation	Prayer
My body's natural intelligence is working in me now to promote health.	God, I know that you are working in me now to promote health.
I know that each day I am closer to having a healthy back.	God, I know that each day you guide me closer to having a healthy back.
My mind can control my comfort level.	God, with your guidance, my mind can control my comfort level.

Some Pointers Before You Start

Don't bargain: Prayer is not bargaining—as in, "God, if you'll do this for me, I promise to be good for the rest of my life." Prayer is simply speaking with a higher power and aligning yourself with positive energy.

Nonspecific prayer works: You do not need to pray for a specific outcome—as in, "God, please heal the left side of my lower back." Rather, pray, "God, please guide me to my good," or " God, I ask for that which is my highest good and the highest good of all other beings."

Prayer is positive energy: The positive energy sent out when praying attracts more positive energy.

Prayer and hope: Though many scientists may be skeptical about the effects of prayer, it cannot hurt. Prayer fosters hope and hope reduces suffering.

Gratitude: Always remember to include some word of thanks in each prayer for the good already received and for the good that is coming.

Anywhere/anytime: Remember you can pray anywhere, anytime, silently in your heart, even if it is only a sentence or two.

Make a sacred space: Consider making a prayer space in the home--a special room or part of a room dedicated to prayer, where you might have a picture, statue, candle, incense, crystals, shells, flowers, stones, or anything else from nature that brings pleasure or reminds you of a higher power. Try to sit in that special prayer space at least once a day.

Consult: A priest, rabbi, or minister can tell you about books of prayers from which to draw or adapt prayers for specific needs and beliefs.

CHAPTER 14

THE USE OF MIND MACHINES TO RELIEVE ANXIETY AND PAIN AND REPROGRAM THE BRAIN FOR HEALING

What Are They?

MIND MACHINES ARE SMALL COMPUTERS that control brain wave activity through various light and sound frequencies. According to the Mindgear Catalog, "through flickering lights and precisely controlled rhythmic tones, [these devices] stimulate and synchronize the hemispheres of the brain while entraining the brain wave frequencies into desirable states of consciousness." Typically these machines come with LED glasses containing four pulsating lights for each eye, stereo headphones to transmit the various rhythmic tones, and also "cranial electrical stimulation" devices that attach to the ears. As described in the Mindgear catalog, "cranial electrical stimulation pulses micro current through electrodes attached to the ears in order to optimize and normalize brain functioning by stimulating parts of the brain that are not functioning at peak performance."

While all of this sounds a bit like science fiction, be assured that mind machines are safe, based on solid research principles, and when used daily can reduce stress and help release endorphins.

How Do They Work?

Without getting too technical, mind machines can assist us in producing various brainwave states at will. By changing the light and sound patterns and frequencies, the user can control the mind and produce very specific brain wave states to achieve physical or emotional healing, academic or athletic excellence, increased learning ability and improved memory. These brainwave states are described below:

• Beta Brain Waves: (13 to 32 and above, cycles per second, or Hz) The awake state, normal alert consciousness. This pattern is conducive to stimulating energy and action; it is optimal for intense mental activities such as calculations, highly structured functions including logical, analytical, intellectual thinking and verbal communication.

• Alpha Brain Waves: (8 to 12 Hz) The relaxed, lucid stage. This pattern is conducive to mood elevation, stress reduction, motivation, inspiration, and intuitive insights. One is relaxed, but yet alert.

• Theta Brain Waves: (4 to 8 Hz) Meditation, deep relaxation, mental imagery and twilight learning stage. This pattern can be viewed as near sleep—brain waves that are conducive to inner peace, physical and emotional healing, and deep unconscious imagery and creativity.

• Delta Brain Waves: (.5 to 4 Hz) Deep dreamless sleep. This pattern is characterized by a slow wave restorative sleep. It is conducive to divine knowledge and miraculous healing, and personal growth.

Mind machines are generally pre-programmed to accomplish certain defined goals. The various pre-programmed sessions deal with such areas as stress management and high performance, insomnia, pain relief, anxiety and panic disorders, conflict resolution, substance abuse, eating disorders, self esteem, confidence, performance enhancement, and learning enhancement. Program sessions vary from 10 to 20 minutes on the average. Cranial electrical stimulation machines generate micro-electrical impulses to the ear lobes, enhancing these sessions and releasing endorphins. Mind machines provide an additional plus—by putting the brain into the theta state, while at the same time listening to a learning audio tape or relaxation audio tape, its effectiveness is enhanced tremendously. Thus, more is remembered or a deeper state of relaxation is achieved.

How Can Mind Machines Assist in Relieving and Healing Pain?
Mind machines can easily place us in a relaxed, meditative state, removing all levels of anxiety. Certainly this alone substantially moderates the pain experience, especially if the pain is psychologically induced. More importantly, there are mind machine programs specifically for pain relief.

In the Voyager XL system, produced by Theta Technologies, there is a pain relief program that operates in conjunction with an audio tape. Light and sound machines can increase endorphin levels. Moreover, in this specific program, a special combination of hypnosis and imagery is used to remove the source of pain through disassociation of the pain from the body, transformation of specific symbols for tension and discomfort and reintegration of a new symbol for resolved tension and synthesis. Through the integrated cassette program, used in conjunction with the Voyager, the session takes the user from a high beta level to a lowered theta level, eventually returning to a low alpha level.

Sources for Mind Machines and Other Related Products

There are at least two companies that produce or market mind machines. Each company is listed below with a brief description of its products.

• **Theta Technologies: (800) 395-9148**

Theta Technologies markets a mind machine entitled "Voyager XL," the mental fitness system. It contains 50 built-in programs, in five categories, including, relax, explore, learn, change and energize. Other audio tapes or CD's can be used in conjunction with the machine. It is extremely simple to operate.

• **Mindgear, Inc.: (800) 525 6463**

Mindgear produces three machines ranging from a low end, to a middle and high end product. Its low-end product, entitled the "SLX Personal Relaxation System," has 16 built-in programs, frequency control, binaural sound, digital display, is adaptable to future software upgrades, and has four stimulation modalities comprising the phasing of the lights and sounds for different effects.

In the middle product, entitled, the "PR-2X System," there are 30 built-in pre-programmed sessions, six stimulation modalities, 5 auto pilot programs that generate an unlimited number of unique sound and light sessions. It can also store autopilot sessions, scale the programs from 5 minutes to two hours, with four selectable tones, and can accommodate two users.

The high end system, the "XCELR8R II," connects to a personal computer, has 50 built in programs, and has all the other features of the PR-2X system. All systems come with stereo headphones, one pair of LED glasses, stereo patch cords and the actual box the headphones and glasses are connected to. This box contains the appropriate chips to control the programs. Mindgear also markets the sound and light turbo charger. This machine sends micro electric currents to the ear lobes, through electrodes.

• **Tools for Exploration: (415) 499-9056**

This mail-order retailer produces an excellent catalog describing various mind machines and other products helpful in relieving pain. Call for a catalog.

While not for everyone, mind machines have proven effective in relieving pain and promoting relaxation and meditation.

CHAPTER 15

FIREWALKING TECHNIQUES TO CONTROL PAIN

THE AUTHORS ARE INDEBTED to Brad Steiger and Komar, who graciously allowed us to use material from their book *Life Without Pain*. Mr. Steiger puts Komar's thoughts into words.

What Is It?

In firewalking, normal, everyday folks, not entranced yogis, walk over burning coals as a sort of rite of passage. It is the ultimate mind-over-matter experience, and the ultimate in pain control because firewalkers walk over burning red hot coals without pain or injury. It is generally taught in a three-hour session. We, of course, are not suggesting walking over burning hot coals as part of a pain management program, *but the principles can be applied to reduce and possibly eliminate back pain.*

Why Does It Work?

The intention to be pain free is the key. Firewalk instructors teach, through a variety of methods, how to harness this intention, so that pain is not felt and injury to the feet does not occur. The method makes use of the strong mind-body connection.

How Do You Do It?

The steps in Komar's five-day program involve the basic principles that underlie all the pain control techniques presented in this book:
• Positive thinking and the power of the mind-body connection
• Relaxation and exercise
• Deep breathing and rhythmic breathing—breathing out twice as long as breathing in (See Chapter 5 for detailed instructions).
• Meditation techniques to promote focus
• Thought substitution

The Five-Day Pain Control Program

Follow the steps carefully and you will have an excellent chance of significantly reducing or eliminating pain. Each day requires only two five-minute sessions. We suggest, as with meditation and self-hypnosis, choosing an appropriate time for these sessions when you can relax, concentrate, and work undisturbed.

Day One: Both sessions on the first day require stating affirmatively that you will not permit pain in your life.

• *The First Five-Minute Session*

1. Designed to relax the body, regulate respiration, and mentally condition you to remove pain from the thinking process.
2. Sit erect in a chair with the back straight and feet flat on the floor.
3. Breathe in deeply, and while doing so, mentally state "I feel."
4. On the exhalation mentally state "no pain."
5. Continue the breathing and mental statements for three minutes.
6. Then drop the head forward onto your chest, roll it to the left, up and over the left shoulder as far back as possible without straining and continue this three more times.
7. Reverse the procedure and lower the head to the chest and roll it to the right, in the same manner as the left, three times.
8. Return to the left three more times and then to the right three more times for a total of two minutes.

• *The Second Five-Minute Session.*

1. Do the head roll in the same sequence as the first session for two minutes.
2. Finish with three minutes of rhythmic breathing, repeating mentally "I feel" on the inhalation and "no pain" on the exhalation.

Day Two:

• *The First Five-Minute Session*

1. Stand straight with heels close together and raise yourself up on the toes, hold for a count of three, then lower onto your heels, and repeat for approximately one minute. Later this is referred to as "heel raises."
2. Follow with about two minutes of head rolls in the same manner as day one.
3. Complete this session with two minutes of rhythmic breathing repeating mentally "I feel" on inhalation and "no pain" on the exhalation.

• *The Second Five-Minute Session*

1. Stand erect, feet comfortably apart and raise your arms over the head and stretch for the ceiling, visualizing the hands flattening against the ceiling. When the tension becomes uncomfortable in the arms, lower them and stretch again. Repeat for two minutes.

2. Do one minute of head rolls.

3. Conclude with two minutes of rhythmic breathing as in the first session of the day mentally stating "I feel" on the inhalation and "no pain" exhalation as before.

Day Three:

• *The First Five-Minute Session*

1. Stretch to the ceiling for one minute as on day two.

2. Follow with one minute of heel raises.

3. Then one minute of head rolls.

4. Conclude with two minutes of rhythmic breathing mentally stating " I feel...no pain" as done on day two.

• *The Second Five-Minute Session*

1. Lie flat on the floor for one minute rhythmically breathing "I feel...no pain".

2. While breathing focus on a painful area in the body. Visualize the painful area as bright red in color and picture in the mind's eye a cool damp cloth in your hand and start rubbing away the area of pain. As the area becomes smaller, visualize the pain leaving forever.

3. Continue this process for four minutes.

4. Conclude the session by rhythmically breathing and stating "I feel...no pain."

Day Four:

• *The First Five-Minute Session*

1. For the first minute, stand erect, raise the arms over the head and bend at the waist to touch the toes. Stretch as far as is comfortable, though it is not necessary to touch the toes. If you cannot do this, sit or stand and contract the stomach muscles for one minute.

2. Rest, and then do one minute of stretching to the ceiling.

3. Then do one minute of head rolls.

4. Rest for a moment and then do one minute of heel raises.

5. Conclude by rhythmically breathing "I feel...no pain" for one minute.

• *The Second Five-Minute Session*
1. Stand before a mirror concentrating on your face.
2. Rhythmically breathe and mentally state " I feel...no pain."
3. Permit your face to have a happy expression.
4. Visualize the pain leaving the body as your smile becomes wider and wider.
5. Continue this process for the full five minutes.

Day Five:
• *The First Five-Minute Session*
1. Stand erect in front of a chair and bend the knees until the buttocks touch the seat of the chair, and then rise to a standing position. Continue these deep knee bends for one minute.
2. Touch toes or contract abdomen for one minute.
3. Do head rolls for one minute.
4. Conclude with heel raises, but as you lift up on the toes mentally recite " I feel" and as you lower the toes mentally recite "no pain." Continue for about two minutes.
•*The Second Five-Minute Session*
1. Stand before a mirror and mentally appraise yourself, noticing how much more relaxed your face looks and also assess how much better your body feels. Pain is leaving your life.
2. While focusing on your smiling face for the full five minutes rhythmically breathe in a joyful manner and mentally state "I feel"on the inhalation and " no pain" on the exhalation.

This technique incorporates many of the mental means of pain relief presented already. We recommend that you give this technique a try and use it in conjunction with the recommended programs.

(Komar can be contacted at P.O. Box 87, Wilmot, OH 44689 / 330-359-5748)

CHAPTER 16

THE EXERCISE PROGRAM

IN EXERCISE WE EXERT THE BODY BY MOVING different parts to make them stronger and more flexible. There are six types of exercises in the program: warm-up, aerobic, strengthening, stretching, specific back exercises, and walking.

Why Does It Work?

Exercise has many benefits. For chronic back pain sufferers it lessens and can eventually eliminate pain. Weak back muscles cause pain because they place a great deal of stress on the spine. Exercise makes muscles more flexible and strong.

Exercise has a number of other benefits for the chronic pain sufferer. Vigorous physical exercise stimulates the production of endorphins, thus relieving pain and improving mood. Exercise also stimulates and energizes you. Aerobic exercise causes the body to take in more oxygen, improves blood circulation, and helps you handle the stress of pain. Strengthening exercises build up muscles so that they better support the spine. Stretching improves the flexibility of your muscles and prevents them from going into spasm. Back exercises are designed to make the specific muscles in and around the back stronger and more flexible. Walking invigorates the whole system, but specifically focuses on the legs, trunk and lower back. Exercising each day, every day, is essential.

How Do You Do It?

The exercise program consists of two levels: 1. beginning and 2. the full workout. *The Beginning Workout:* This is designed for those who have not been on a regular exercise program. It is gentle and consists of the following steps:
1. A gentle warm-up
2. Special gentle strengthening and toning exercises
3. Stretching
4. Back Exercises
5. Walking

The Full Workout: This workout is for the most part the one author Miller followed at the beginning of his treatment at Stanford's Pain Management Center. It is somewhat challenging and consists of the following steps:

1. Warm-up
2. Aerobic Exercise
3. Strengthening Exercises
4. Stretching Exercises
5. Back Exercises
6. Walking

Whichever routine you choose, it should be done daily, except that the strengthening and aerobic exercises are done every other day in either workout.

Instructions Before Exercising—Read Carefully

Discuss the exercise programs with your physician, and obtain his/her clearance before commencing either one. Certain of the recommended exercises may not be compatible with your condition. However, all of the exercises are consistent with a normal back pain exercise program.

Start slowly. While many of the exercises will call for a specific number of repetitions, or amount of time to exercise, these are the maximums recommended. For example in aerobics, work up to 20 minutes, starting with 5, then 10, then 15 and finally 20 minutes. In strengthening exercises, while the maximum repetitions will be 30, start slowly with 5, then 10, then 15, then 20 and then 30. With stretching, while many stretches are to be held until the count of 20, in the beginning hold until 10 and then work your way up. Experiment with the back exercises, doing them slowly and gently and making sure none aggravates your condition. If an increase of 5 minutes in aerobics or of 5 repetitions in strengthening exercises induces pain, then scale back and increase by one minute in aerobics and 1 or 2 repetitions in other exercises. While the walking program will eventually require two miles a day, build up to this slowly, walking only a block in the beginning. It is very important to start slowly as many of you have not exercised for significant periods of time. If it hurts, slow down, though it is normal to feel some soreness in the beginning.

Follow the written instructions precisely after reviewing the illustrations showing the basic position and suggested movements. Proper deep breathing is important. As a general rule, you breathe in before exerting effort and exhale when exerting effort.

Listen to your body. While some mild soreness is expected when you commence exercising, if real pain develops or persists, cease the exercises and discuss what is happening with your doctor or physical therapist.

Do exercise, do not skip a day, unless you are otherwise sick. Remember this is an investment, one that will pay off in terms of pain reduction, mood elevation, and improved quality of life.

THE BEGINNING AND GENTLE WORKOUT

This consists of a warm-up, special strengthening exercises, certain of the stretches and back exercises in the full workout and walking. The gentle workout will be described by type of exercise. Reference at times will be made to some of the exercises specified in the full workout section.

The Warm-up

This is designed to get the blood flowing in your system and gently loosen stiff muscles. It is vitally important that you do this warm-up prior to commencing the beginning or full workout. The exercises are a combination of movements from traditional Western and Eastern chi gung exercises. If you have been inactive for some time and are very stiff, take a warm shower and/or use a moist heating pad on your back before doing the warm up.

The Warm-Up Exercises

Arm Circles:
Purpose: To start blood circulation in the upper trunk.
Repetitions: 15 circles in each direction.
Starting Position: Stand erect with your arms at sides.
Movements:
1. Lift both arms up so that they are perpendicular to body.
2. Start circling arms in a counter clock wise direction for a total of 15 times gradually increasing the diameter of the circle you make with hands form 0 inches to 10 inches.
3. Reverse direction to clockwise and circle arms so that the diameter of the

circle is lessening to 0 inches.

4. Lower hands.

Final Position: Standing erect with arms at your side.

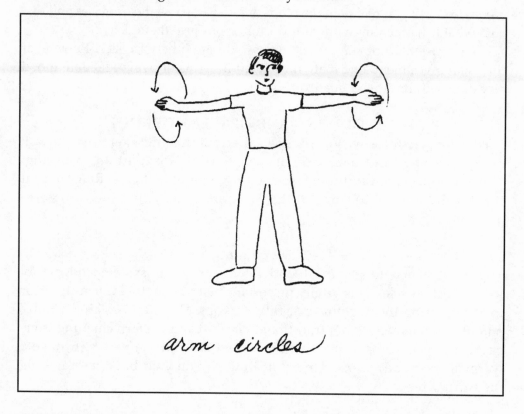

arm circles

Marching in Place:

Purpose: To circulate blood and loosen muscles throughout the body.

Repetitions: Take 100 steps and move arms forward and back in cadence with your steps.

Starting Position: Standing erect with arms down by sides.

Movements:

1. Lift left leg and foot off the floor, about 6 inches while moving right arm forward about 6 inches.

2. Return left foot to the floor and raise right foot up about six inches while moving left arm forward about 6 inches and return left arm next to body.

3. Repeat process 50 times for each foot.

Final Position: Standing erect with arms down by sides.

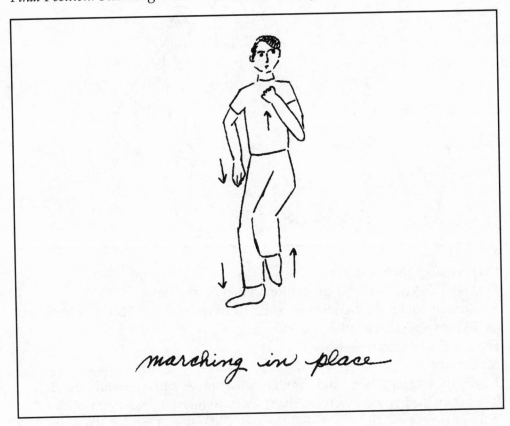

marching in place

Knee Circles:

Purpose: To circulate blood in and loosen muscles in lower extremities.

Repetitions: Circle 25 times to the right and 25 times to the left.

Starting Position: Standing erect.

Movements:

1. Lean over and place hands on knees and bend knees.

2. Place knees together and with hands on knees circle knees 25 times in a clockwise turning movement.

3. Then circle 25 times counter clockwise with hands on knees.

Final Position: Stand erect.

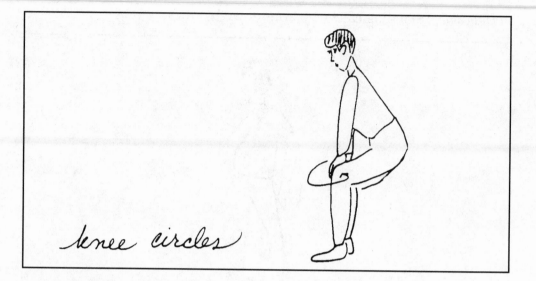

knee circles

Shaking the Hands and Feet:

Purpose: To increase blood circulation in hands and feet.

Repetitions: Shake the hands and arms 10 times out and 10 times back and shake the feet 5 times out and back.

Starting Position: Stand erect.

Movements:

1. Start shaking each hand and simultaneously raise both arms and extend them 2 feet from the body and return. Shake them 10 times in and 10 times back.

2. Then raise your right foot slightly and shake it and the leg ten times, put back in place and do the same with left foot and leg.

Final Position: Standing erect as in the starting position.

Shaking the hands and feet

Full Body Tapping:

Purpose: To awaken the vital life energy in the body.

Repetitions: 7 taps on each side of the arms and legs and 7 taps on each side of the trunk. Repeat two more times.

Starting Position: Stand erect with hands by sides drawn in fists.

Movements:

1. Place right hand on the left side of belly button and tap up trunk to left shoulder for 7 times, then tap 7 times down the inside of left arm. Then tap

from wrist on the outside of the arm up to the shoulder. Repeat two more times.

2. Place left hand on the right side of belly button and tap up trunk to right shoulder for 7 times, tap 7 times down the inside of right arm, and then 7 times from wrist on the outside of the arm to the right shoulder. Repeat 2 more times.

3. Place your left hand on the outside at the top of the left leg and tap 14 times down to outer ankle, then tap up the inside of left leg 14 times up to waist. Repeat 2 more times.

4. Place right hand on the outside at the top of the right leg and tap 14 times down to your outer ankle, then tap up the inside of right leg 14 times up to the waist. Repeat 2 more times.

5. Place each fist on either side of the spine about 2 inches away from it at the waist and tap up to the mid back and tap back down to waist 7 times. Move fist out another 2 inches and tap up to mid back and back to waist again 7 times. Repeat entire process 2 more times.

Final Position: Standing erect.

Full body tapping

Tap sides of arms, trunk, and legs

Tap from belly button up to shoulder and down inside of arm on each side

Bending Knees And Tapping Hips:

Purpose: To circulate chi and blood in the body.

Repetitions: Slightly bend knees and then raise knees 200 times and tap sides of thighs 200 times.

Starting Position: Stand erect with hands by sides.

Movements:

1. Gently bend knees about 6 inches and at same time tap outside thighs with open hands.
2. Return to starting position.
3. Repeat 199 more times.

Final Position: Same as starting position.

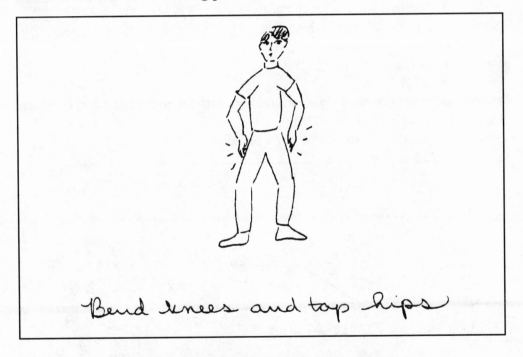

Bend knees and tap hips

The Special Strengthening Exercises

These exercises were taught to author Miller by Andrew Morris, a Touch For Health instructor and faculty member at the World School of Massage and Advanced Healing Arts. They effectively strengthen, balance and tone muscles with little stress or strain on the body.

Each exercise should be done in a rhythm of 2 seconds upward and 2 seconds downward motion. The stimulation points are rubbed on both sides of the body to enhance muscular response to the exercises. Rub these points with your index fingers for about 30-45 seconds. Do 2 repetitions of each exercise and then rub the points.

The Bent Leg Raise:
Purpose: To strengthen the psoas muscle.
Repetitions: 2 times each leg.
Starting Position: Lying on back, legs straight, arms by your side, head on floor.
Movements:
1. Lift right leg, keeping foot higher than knee, bringing it up until thigh makes a 110 degree angle with the body. Then lower leg.
2. Do the same movement with left leg.
3. Repeat the movements again.
Final Position: Lying on your back.
Point Stimulation:
1. Massage points on both sides of navel located one inch above and one inch from navel.
2. Massage points at ends of right and left ribs.

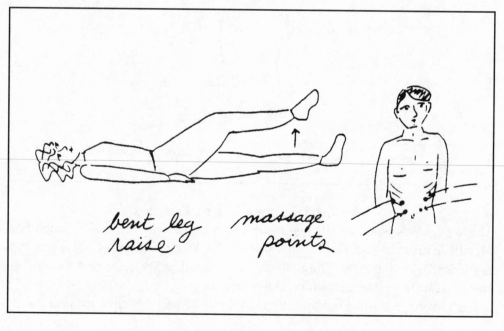

bent leg raise   massage points

Straight Arm Pullovers:

Purpose: To strengthen the pectorals.

Repetitions: Two times.

Starting Position: Lay on your back with the knees bent and feet out wider than the hips.

Movements:

1. Raise your right arm straight up so that wrist is directly above the eyes. Then lower arm.

2. Do same movement with left arm.

3. Repeat movements again.

Final Position: Same as starting position.

Point Stimulation: Massage the sore points about one inch directly under both nipples.

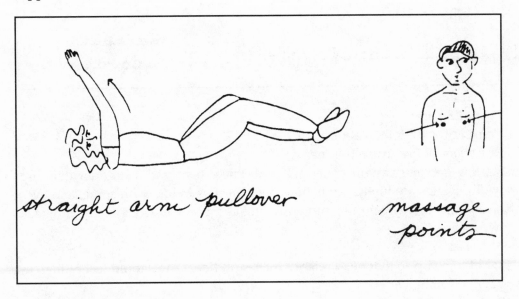

straight arm pullover

massage points

Partial Push-Offs

Purpose: To strengthen pectoral muscles and arms.

Repetitions: Two times.

Starting Position: Lay on belly, legs relaxed, hands even with ears and palms on the floor.

Movements:

1. Direct your pressure into the floor and raise upper trunk 6 inches off the floor.

2. Gently lower your weight on your hands so that hands bear the weight not your back.

3. Repeat again.

Final Position: Same as starting position.

Point Stimulation: Massage the sore points about once inch below the nipples.

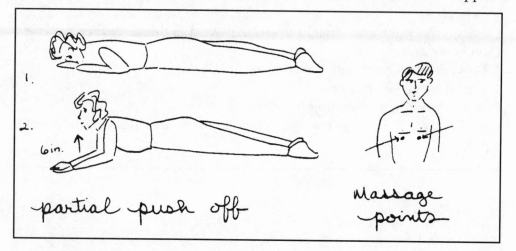

partial push off

Massage points

Partial Sit-up:

Purpose: To strengthen abdominals.

Repetitions: Raise trunk 10 times.

Starting Position: Lay on your back with knees bent and feet wider than hip width. Hands are interlaced behind neck, neck is in line with spine, and eyes on a point slightly behind point on ceiling as if you were looking up and back two inches.

Movements:

1. Lift torso up so that head raises 2 inches off floor. You should feel pulling in your abdominal area.

2. Lower head and torso.

3. Repeat 9 more times.

Final Position: Same as starting position.

Point Stimulation:

1. Sit up and cross legs.

2. Rub points on inside of thigh from knee to 2/3rds of the way up the thigh.

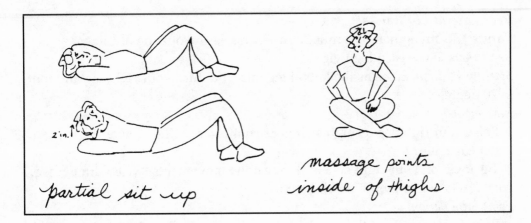

partial sit up

massage points
inside of thighs

Lateral Leg Raises:
Purpose: To strengthen the buttocks muscles.
Repetitions: Raise and lower each leg 2 times.
Starting Position: Lay on left side with head propped in your left hand and left leg bent 90 degrees. Knees and shoulders and hips face left.
Movements:
1. Raise right leg as high as it goes comfortably without rotating.
2. Then lower right leg and repeat.
3. Turn over onto right side and raise left leg in the same manner as in step 1 and repeat.
Final Position: Same as starting position.
Point Stimulation: Place index and middle fingers of both hands on top of pubic bone and massage across top of pubic bone.

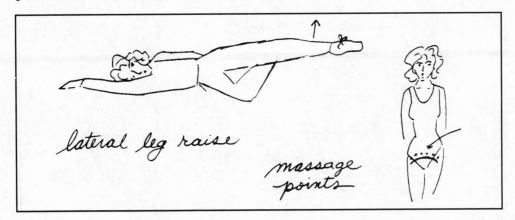

lateral leg raise

massage
points

Rear Lateral Leg Raises:

Purpose: To strengthen butt muscles and muscles on outside of thighs.

Repetitions: Raise each leg twice.

Starting Position: Same as the lateral leg raise, but turn your right leg and foot in 20 degrees.

Movements:

1. Raise your right leg as high as it goes comfortably. Then lower the leg.

2. Repeat again.

3. Turnover on your right side and repeat the movements twice with left leg.

Final Position: Lying on your right side.

Point Stimulation:

1. Rub points on top of thigh to knee.

2. Rub points on outside of thigh from hip bone to knee.

rear lateral leg raise

massage points
1. top of thigh
   to knee
2. side of thigh
   from hip bone
   to knee

Upper Back Toner:
Purpose: To loosen and strengthen upper back.
Repetitions: Twice.
Starting Position: Lay on belly looking down at floor with legs relaxed with arms at sides.
Movements:
1. Raise chest from floor about 6 inches while hands reach back facing towards each other and shoulders pulled down and back relative to head. Breathe out on lifting. Pull up gently. This should be felt in upper back.
2. Repeat one more time.
Final Position: Same as starting position.
Point Stimulation: On left side only stimulate the point about 2 inches below the nipple on the rib cage.

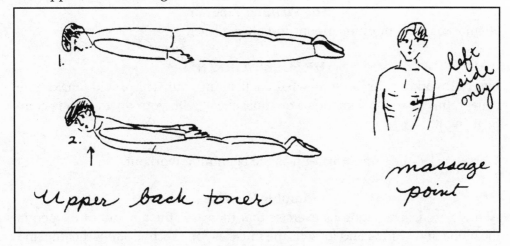

Upper back toner

massage point

left side only

The Stretches
Important: Be sure to read the general instructions for stretching later in this chapter before doing these exercises and follow them carefully.
Do the following stretches in the order listed below. The instructions for these can be found in the Stretching Section of the full workout.
1. Calf Stretch-2 times
2. Quadriceps-Stretch-2 times
3. Standing Side Stretch-1 time
4. Hip Flexor Stretch-1 time

5. Upper and Mid Back Stretch-1 time
6. Conservative Hamstring Stretch-2 times

The Back Exercises

Do the following back exercises in the order listed below. The instructions for these can be found in the Back Exercise section of the full workout.
1. Pelvic Tilt-5 times
2. Knee to Chest-1 time
3. Quadruped Stretch-5 times
4. Prone Extension-5 times
5. Back Release-5 times
6. Elbow Press-up-2 times

The Walking Program

20 minute walks morning, noon, and after dinner.

THE FULL WORKOUT

The full workout can be somewhat challenging, but will provide maximum benefit. In view of its demands, you must check with your doctor before commencing it.

Warm-up: Do the same warm-up as the beginning workout.

Aerobic Exercise

Aerobic exercise is vigorous exercise that increases the amount of oxygen in the blood and warms and loosens the muscles for effective strengthening and stretching. If you lift light weights or stretch unwarmed or tight muscles, minor muscle tears will result and pain levels will increase.

After you work up to it, you should do 20 minutes of aerobic exercise at 70%-80% of your maximum heart rate. Do not go over 80% of your maximum heart rate. Here is the formula for calculating this:

220-your age x .70 = 70% of your maximum heart rate

So, for a 45-year old person the calculations would look like this:

220-45=175   175 x .70 = 122 (beats per minute)

Thus, a 45-year old needs to get his/her heart rate up to 122 beats per minute to be exercising at 70% of maximum.

While exercising you can check your heart rate with a monitor. They cost between $75 and $100. Alternatively you can take your pulse while exercising for 15 seconds and multiply it by 4 to calculate your heart rate.

A stationary bike or treadmill can provide aerobic-level exercise. We recommend purchasing an electric treadmill with a speedometer and that can be elevated. Many have an ear attachment which will also show the heart rate while exercising. These treadmills, which cost between $300 and $400, are worth the investment, because you can do the required aerobic exercise in your home in any type of weather. Build up slowly to exercising for 20 minutes at 70-80% of your maximum heart rate. Start with 5 minutes gradually building up to 20 minutes. In all probability you will need to walk briskly on the treadmill at a speed of about 3.7- 4.0 miles per hour at a slight elevation. You will be sweating at least half way through the workout. Enjoy the exercise by placing the treadmill or bicycle in front of a TV and watch a favorite comedy show.

You should engage in an aerobic workout at least every other day. As you build up to the 20 minutes, you will begin to release endorphins.

You must discuss your intended aerobic exercise with your physician. If you are over 35, your doctor will probably test your heart with an EKG, to see if you can withstand this form of vigorous exercise. If you cannot do 20 minutes on a treadmill or stationary bike for medical reasons, have your physician suggest some form of safe effective aerobic exercise.

The Strengthening Exercises

Do the special strengthening exercises detailed in the Beginning and Gentle Workout section.

Additional strengthening exercises are identified below. The starting position, a step-by-step written instruction on the movements, the finishing position, proper breathing and pictures of starting positions and progress through the exercise, and number of repetitions are detailed.

In the beginning use two hand held 1.5 pound light weights. These can be purchased at any sporting goods store. If, after a number of weeks, you feel you can lift more, increase the weight to 2.5 pounds per weight. There is no need to go higher than that.

The Triceps Strengthener:
Repetitions: 30 on each side.

Starting Position: Lie on back with your feet flat on the floor, knees bent.
Movements:

1. Place both weights in right hand.
2. Lift the right arm up so that it is perpendicular to body.
3. Place left hand under right elbow for support.
4. Slowly bend right arm at the elbow, until right hand comes within 2 inches of shoulder.
5. Slowly raise the right forearm to a straight position and bend at elbow again.
6. After doing 10 repetitions, move the weight to the left arm, repeat the process ten times, and return the weight to the right arm and continue the process 2 more sets of 10 each.

Final Position: Left arm straight with weight in hand.
Breathing: Breathe in as you bring weights down; breathe out when you lift weights up.

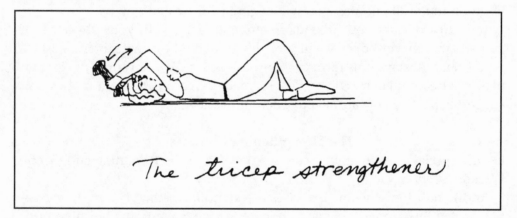

The tricep strengthener

The Pectoral Strengthener:
Repetitions: 30
Starting Position: Lie on back, with feet flat and knees bent.
Movements:

1. Place one weight in each hand and raise arms so that they are straight, perpendicular to the body and both weights are touching each other in the air.
2. Keeping arms straight, move left arm out to the left, right arm out to the right, until both arms are at a 45 degree angle to your body.

3. Keeping both arms straight, return them to the starting position.

4. Repeat the movements 29 times.

Final Position: Both arms will be straight in the air, with the weights touching each other.

Breathing: Breathe in as arms go down, and breathe out when arms are being raised.

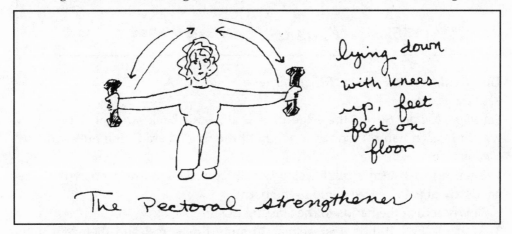

The Pectoral strengthener

lying down with knees up, feet flat on floor

The Shoulder Strengtheners:

Repetitions: 30 each side.

Starting Position: Lie on back with feet flat and knees bent. Roll over on right side with right arm away from the body. Pick up the two weights with left arm and place left elbow on left hip with hand on the floor.

Movements:

1. Keeping left elbow on hip and forearm straight, lift the weights off the ground so that the hand is at a 45 degree angle to the body, above the left hip.

2. Slowly return the left hand to the starting position.

3. After 10 repetitions, rest, do 10 more repetitions, rest and then complete the final 10 repetitions.

4. Turn over on the left side and repeat the process with the weights in the right hand, after assuming the above described position.

5. Remember to rest after each 10 repetitions.

Final Position: On left side with the weights in right hand.

Breathing: As you lower the weights to the floor breathe in, and exhale as you raise the weights off the ground.

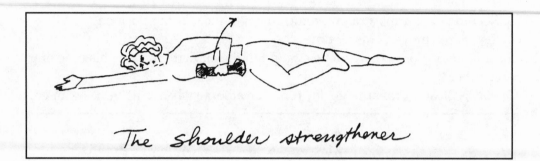

The shoulder strengthener

The Shoulder and Forearm Strengtheners:

Repetitions: 30

Starting Position: Sit on the edge of a chair, with back straight. Grasp one weight in each hand. Turn wrists so that little fingers are facing outward.

Movements:

1. Keeping each arm straight, slowly raise the weights to a point that the hands are at a 45 degree angle to the body.

2. Slowly return the hands to the starting position.

3. After the first 10 lifts, rest, repeat 10 more times, rest and then repeat 10 more times.

Final Position: Sitting on the chair with weights in each hand, hands by the sides.

Breathing: As you lower arms to the sides breathe in; as you raise arms, breathe out.

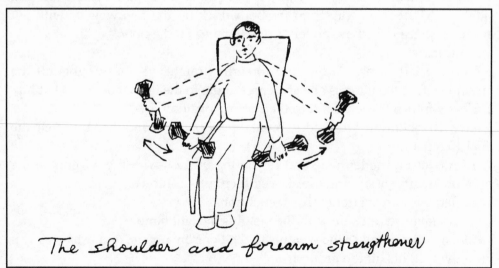

The shoulder and forearm strengthener

The Biceps Strengthener:

Repetitions: 30 times each side.

Starting Position: Sitting straight in a chair, put both weights in right hand, with arms at sides.

Movements:

1. Lift right forearm up slowly with the weights in right hand, while bending the arm at the elbow. Raise forearm so that the weight comes within five inches of the shoulder.

2. Return the right forearm to the starting position.

3. After ten repetitions, move the weights to your left hand and do 10 repetitions as in step 1. Do 2 more sets of 10 repetitions on each arm, alternating from right to left between sets.

Final Position: Sitting with weights in left hand, with left arm straight down.

Breathing: Breathe in when lowering weights and breathe out when lifting.

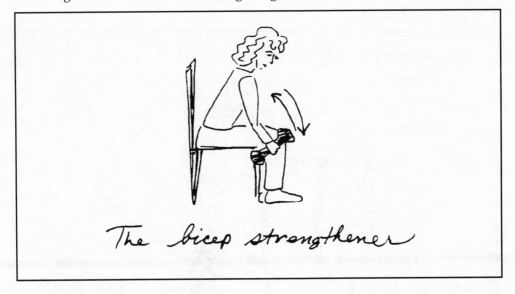

The bicep strengthener

The Leg and Hip Strengtheners:

For this exercise you will need to purchase two 2.5 pound ankle weights which you can strap to each ankle.

Repetitions: 30 each side.

Starting Position: After weights are strapped to each ankle, stand up with your left hand grabbing onto an object that is shoulder height to give you support.

Place feet together.

Movements:

1. With both knees unlocked and legs straight, move the right leg out to the right about 2 and 1/2 feet so that the right foot is at about a 10 degree angle from your body.

2. Return the right foot to the starting position and repeat the process 9 more times.

3. After completing 10 movements with your right leg, grab onto the object with your right hand, and move the left foot out about 2 and 1/2 feet so that the left foot is about a 10 degree angle to your body.

4. Do two more sets of 10 with each leg alternating from right to left.

Final Position: You finish with both feet together and the right hand grabbing onto a shoulder high object.

Breathing: Breathe in as the feet return to the starting position and exhale as you move the feet out.

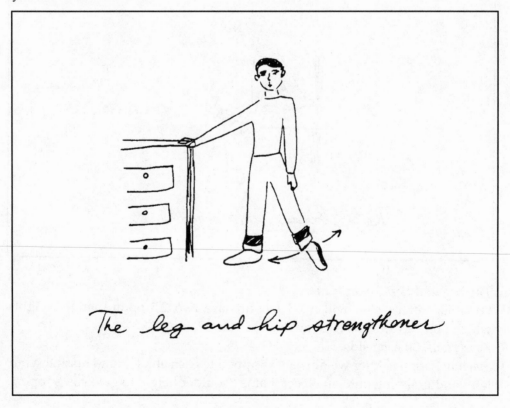

The leg and hip strengthener

The Stretching Exercises

Stretching is a vital component of the exercise program. In *Stretching*, by Bob Anderson, a book which should be in your library, the author notes the following benefits of stretching and suggests how and when to stretch. Study this section carefully. Improper stretching can actually increase your pain levels and possibly increase muscle damage.

Stretching Benefits You Because It:

- Relaxes your mind and body.
- Increases your range of motion.
- Reduces tension in your muscles.
- Prepares your muscles for strenuous activities.
- Increases blood circulation.
- Helps you develop body awareness.
- Loosens tight muscles and eventually reduces muscle spasms.

How Does One Stretch?

Anderson gives the following advice: "The right way (to stretch) is a relaxed, sustained stretch with your attention focused on the muscles being stretched. The wrong way is to bounce up and down, or to stretch to the point of pain. Proper stretching can relieve pain."

There are two levels of a stretch: the easy stretch and then the developmental stretch. Each stretch will be broken down into those two phases.

The easy stretch: In this portion of the stretch you spend 10-15 seconds. Do not bounce, but stretch to the point where a "mild" tension is felt and then relax as you hold the stretch for the balance of the easy portion of the stretch, during which the tension should subside. If it does not, then ease up and find the point of the stretch that is comfortable. The easy stretch reduces the tightness of the muscles and prepares them for the developmental stretch.

The developmental stretch: Once the easy portion of the stretch is completed, move into the developmental portion of the stretch. Press forward in the stretch until you feel a mild tension and hold for 20-30 seconds. If tension does not diminish, ease off slightly. This portion of the stretch tones the muscles and increases flexibility.

Breathing: Breathe in as you are holding the stretch and exhale when moving into the stretch. The breathing needs to be slow, controlled, and rhythmi-

145

cal. Do not hold your breath while stretching.

Counting: Count slowly to yourself by stating one and two and three etc. until you hold the stretch for the required time.

Avoid Improper Stretching: If you bounce or stretch too far you will activate the "stretch reflex," which is a nerve reflex that signals the muscles to contract and tighten up. Improper stretching can cause microscopic tears in the muscles eventually leading to the formation of scar tissue. At this point you develop sore and tight muscles. Proper stretching should not cause pain. Listen to your body and follow the instructions as written, moving into the easy stretch, then slowly the developmental stretch. Stretch to 70% of the full stretch if you can. If you cannot, then stretch only to the point of comfort until you become more flexible with practice.

When To Stretch

Stretching must be done as a part of the beginning and full workout. We also suggest these stretches be done at least once, but preferably twice a day, at your convenience. Make sure the muscles are warm before stretching. We recommend stretching after showering in the morning and before dinner. Anderson suggests that stretching be done when you are stiff, at different times during the day while TV watching, after sitting or talking for lengthy periods, and while at work to relieve tension. Proper stretching is a necessity for any chronic back pain sufferer. If you don't stretch, you will not relieve pain and stiffness.

The Stretches:

The Calf Stretch:
Purpose: To make the calf muscles more flexible so that your legs can bear more of the weight and strain of walking, pushing and bending.
Repetitions: Two repetitions on right and left calves.
Starting Position: Face a wall, with both hands flat against the wall in line with your shoulders. Place right foot directly behind your left foot about 18 inches and bend the left knee with right foot flat on the ground.
Movements:
1. While remaining in the starting position, bend the front leg forward and move into the easy part of the stretch for 15 seconds, then move into the developmental part of the stretch for 20 seconds. Then ease off. Make sure your

back is flat and both feet are flat on the ground.

2. Change your position so that your right leg is slightly bent, place your left leg and left foot about 18 inches behind your right foot. Bend the right leg forward and move into the easy stretch for 15 seconds, then into the developmental portion of the stretch for another 20 seconds. Then ease off. Make sure your back is flat and both feet are flat on the ground.

3. Change your position to that described in step 1, hold the stretch in the same manner and change positions so that left leg is bent with right foot behind the left foot. Hold the stretch for the period of time indicated in step 2. Repeat the stretch as described in number 2.

Final Position: Your right leg is bent with your left foot behind your right leg.

Helpful Hints: Keep your back heel on the floor. Do not arch your back.

Breathing: Breathe in while holding the stretch, and exhale as you are moving into the stretch.

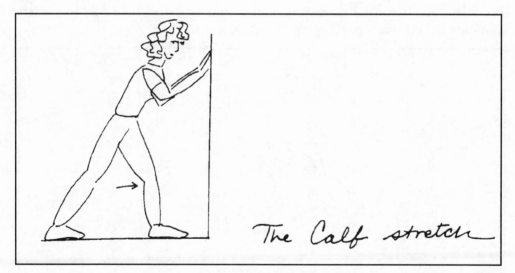

The Calf stretch

The Quadriceps Stretch:

Purpose: To stretch and lengthen muscles in the front of the thigh.

Repetitions: 4 total stretches, 2 on right and 2 on left quad muscles.

Starting Position: Stand facing a wall, place left hand flat against a wall and position your body an arm's length from the wall.

Movements:

1. Lift right leg up and grab the top of right ankle with right hand.

2. Gently pull up right leg and move into the easy stretch, which you will feel in the top of your right thigh, for 15 seconds; then move into the developmental stretch for another 20 seconds.

3. Ease off and then change positions so that right hand is touching the wall, with the right arm extended an arm's length from the body. Then grab your left ankle with your left hand, pull up your leg and move into the easy stretch on the left quad muscle for 15 seconds, then move into the developmental stretch for 20 more seconds by pulling further up on your left ankle.

4. Repeat the process one more time, so that a total of 4 stretches are done, 2 on each leg.

Final Position: You will be facing the wall with right hand on the wall and left hand grabbing your left ankle.

Helpful Hints: Do not twist your back to reach your leg. Do not arch your back.

Breathing: Breathe in while resting against the wall and holding the stretch and breathe out when pulling into the stretch.

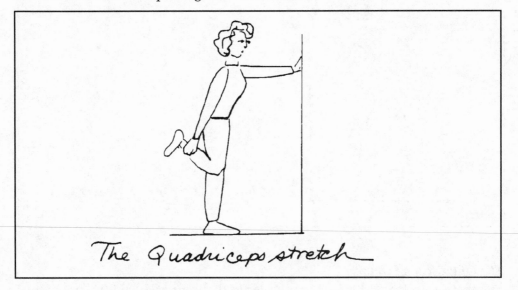

The Quadriceps stretch

The Standing Side Stretch:

Purpose: To stretch the sides of the trunk.

Repetitions: Two stretches on each side.

Starting Position: Stand up straight, with feet directly under hips; then move right arm straight up over your head with right palm facing outward. Knees are slightly bent.

Movements:

1. Bend from waist to the left side so that right hand is at a 30 degree angle to the left side of your body for 15 seconds into the easy stretch, then move your right arm and your waist slightly further to bend into the developmental stretch for an additional 20 seconds.

2. After the stretch is complete, return to the starting position, lower right arm and raise your left arm over your head so that the left palm is facing outward.

3. Repeat the process by bending to your right at the waist until your left hand is at a 30 degree angle to the right side of your body for 15 seconds into the easy stretch; then move right arm and your waist slightly further to the right to bend into the developmental stretch for an additional 20 seconds. Return to the starting position.

4. Repeat steps 1 to 3.

Final Position: Standing straight with your left arm and hand in the air.

Helpful Hints: Do not twist or lift the heels from the floor. Bend from the side, do not twist your trunk.

Breathing: Breathe in while standing with arms in the air and breathe out while moving into the stretch and holding.

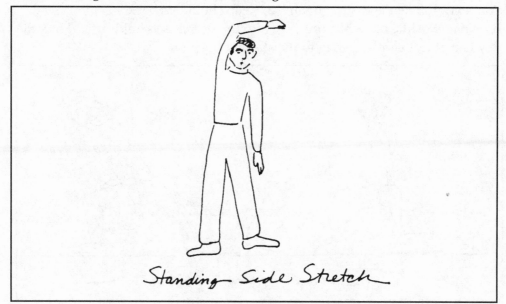

Standing Side Stretch

The Hip Flexor Stretch:

Purpose: To stretch and lengthen the muscles that keep the pelvis and back stable.
Repetitions: 2 on each side.
Starting Position: Kneel on the floor with the right foot extended, right knee bent so that the right leg is at a 90 degree angle to your body. Your left leg and foot are behind with the left leg slightly bent at the knee. Keep back straight and abdominal muscles tightened.
Movements:
1. Lean forward keeping your head straight, moving into the easy stretch for 15 seconds; then move forward into the developmental stretch for another 20 seconds.
2. Ease off the stretch, then switch positions so that the left knee and leg are in front, left knee bent, and right leg bent behind as in movement one. Lean forward towards the left knee, keeping your head straight, moving into the easy stretch for 15 seconds, then move forward in the developmental stretch for another 20 seconds.
3. Ease off, change positions and do two more stretches, one on each side.
Final Position: You will end up with your left knee bent and your right leg and right foot out behind you.
Helpful Hints: Do not arch your back. Do not put your head forward. Keep your eyes focused and straight ahead. Keep shoulders back.
Breathing: Breathe out while pressing into the stretch and holding and breathe in when at rest and returning to the starting position.

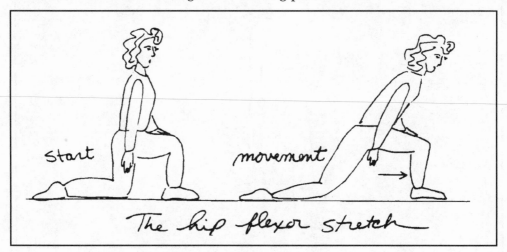

start   movement

The hip flexor stretch

The Upper and Mid Back Stretch:

Purpose: To lengthen and make more supple the muscles of the mid and upper back.

Repetitions: 2 stretches.

Starting Position: Stand straight with both feet shoulder width apart. Grasp hands behind the back so fingers are grabbing each other with left and right palms facing away from the body. Raise both arms so your hands are at mid-back level if possible.

Movements:

1. Gently straighten both arms and move shoulders back and stretch into the easy stretch for 15 seconds and them move the arms and shoulders further back and gently stretch forward into the developmental stretch for another 20 seconds. Bend slightly at the waist while doing this stretch.

2. Return to starting position.

3. Repeat one more time.

Final Position: Same position as starting position.

Helpful Hints: Keep the back flat, do not arch it.

Breathing: Breathe out as you move into the stretch and breathe in as you return.

Upper and mid-back stretch

The Hip Rotator Stretch:

Purpose: This stretch lengthens and strengthens the muscles in and around the hip.

Repetitions: One stretch on each side.

Starting Position: Lie on your back with both feet flat on the floor and knees bent. Place the left leg and foot on the right leg, with the left ankle about 4 inches below the right knee on your thigh and reaching through your legs, grasp with towel or hands the back of the right thigh.

Movements:

1. Gently pull right knee towards you for about 15 seconds into the easy stretch and then move into the developmental stretch for another 20 seconds. Ease off and return to the starting position. You feel the stretch in the right leg that is being pulled back.

2. Switch positions, so that the left knee is bent and the right leg is crossed over the left leg with the right ankle about 4 inches below the left knee. Reaching through your legs with your hands or a towel, grasp the back of the left thigh. Pull the back of the left thigh into the easy stretch for 15 seconds and then move into the developmental stretch for another 20 seconds.

3. Ease off.

Final Position: The left knee is bent with the right leg crossed over the left leg.

Helpful Hints: Keep the neck supported by a pillow. Make sure there is no bounce in the movement. Keep your back flat on the floor. Do not arch it.

Breathing: Exhale as you move into the stretch and inhale as you ease off the stretch. Do not hold your breath.

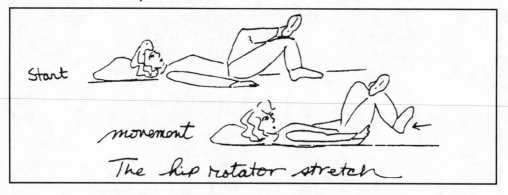

Start

movement

The hip rotator stretch

The Hamstring Stretch

The hamstring stretch is the most important of the stretches because tight hamstrings are one of the predominant causes of low back pain. We are going to suggest three ways to do this stretch. Try each out and see which feels better. Practice this stretch very slowly because you will be stretching muscles in the back as well.

The Conservative Hamstring Stretch:

Purpose: To stretch and loosen hamstring tightness.

Repetitions: Stretch right and left hamstrings twice each in a session.

Starting Position: Stand facing a low stair or stool with body erect, place right heel onto low stool or step, keeping right leg straight, but do not lock your knees.

Movements:

1. Keep the back straight, lift the chest and bend forward from the hips until you feel the stretch in the back of your right thigh. Move into the easy stretch for 15 seconds and then into the developmental stretch for another 20 seconds. Ease off and return to the starting position.

2. Switch sides, with left heel on the low step or stool, left leg straight, and bend from the hip until you feel the stretch in the back of your left thigh. Press forward for 15 seconds of the easy stretch and press further forward for 20 seconds of the developmental stretch.

3. Ease off and repeat the process two more times.

Final Position: Finish with the left heel on the low step or stool in the starting position for that side.

Helpful Hints: Keep the back straight. Do not stretch too far. If you do you can injure your hamstring muscle. Stretch only to a mild point of tension.

Breathing: Breathe in as you are returning from the stretch and exhale as you are moving into and holding the stretch.

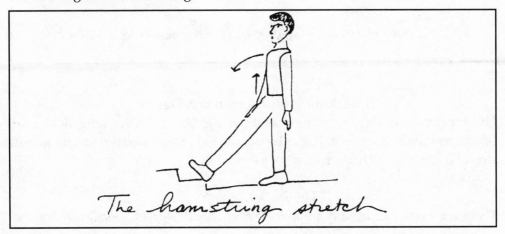

The hamstring stretch

The More Difficult Hamstring Stretch:
Repetitions: 2 stretches on each hamstring muscle.
Starting Position: Lie on your back with your knees bent and arms by your sides.
Movements:
1. Slowly raise right leg with the knee straight. If you are having trouble doing this, you can place a towel around the bottom of the right foot to pull the leg up. Move it up into an easy stretch for 15 seconds and then 20 more seconds in the developmental stretch. Go very slowly at first and at the first sign of strain ease off.
2. Return to the starting position. Now raise your left leg slowly up and hold it into the easy stretch for 15 seconds and then move into the developmental stretch for another 20 seconds
3. Ease off and repeat the process one more time.
Final Position: Lying on the floor with both knees bent.
Breathing: Breathe out as you move forward and hold the stretch and breathe in as you are easing off the stretch.

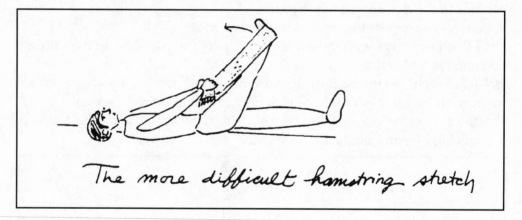

The more difficult hamstring stretch

Stretching With A Prostretch Device

The Prostretch device, retailing for about $29.95, is a stretching device in which you place your foot. It can be purchased at your local sporting goods store. Follow the instructions that come with it.

The Back Exercises

There are a number of very important exercises designed specifically for the back, but which are neither strictly stretching or strengthening. Most are good for you, though some may aggravate an existing condition. We will place a cautionary note where appropriate. Experiment with these exercises, but if one irritates you, eliminate it.

The Pelvic Tilt:

Purpose: To stretch muscles of the low back and to strengthen buttock and stomach muscles.

Repetitions: Start with 3 and work up to 10.

Starting Position: Lie on back with knees bent, feet and hands flat on the floor.

Movements:

1. Tighten the stomach and buttocks muscles and very gently and slowly press the lower back into the floor.

2. Hold position for a count of 5 and release, moving gently back to the starting position.

3. Repeat process 2 more times and gradually work up to 10 pelvic tilts.

Final Position: Same as starting position.

Helpful Hints: Do not jerk or bounce. Do the movement slowly; do not press your back into the floor with a snap or jerk. If it is hard to press the back into the floor, do not press all the way; just go to the point of resistance.

Breathing: Exhale when tail bone is going down and inhale when tailbone is moving up.

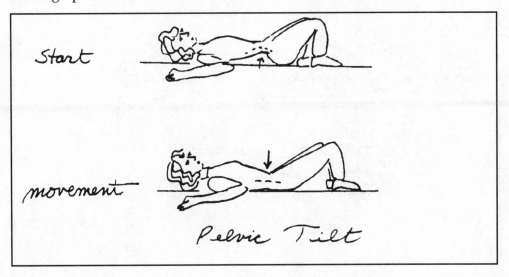

Start

movement

Pelvic Tilt

The Partial Sit-up or Crunches:

Purpose: To strengthen the abdominal muscles, so that you build a strong abdominal muscle brace to support your back.

Repetitions: Start with 5 and work up to 30 per session.

Starting Position: Lie on back with both knees bent and feet flat on the floor, arms crossed over chest with right hand on left shoulder and left hand on right shoulder.

Movements:

1. Look at a point in the ceiling and keep eyes fixed on that point.
2. Tighten the abdominal muscles.
3. Slowly lift shoulder blades off the floor and raise them no higher than 30 degrees. Hold for 3 seconds.
4. Slowly lie back down.
5. Slowly repeat the process 4 more times working up to 30 repetitions.

Final Position: Lying on your back in the starting position.

Helpful Hints: Do not pull up with your neck; keep it relaxed. Keep your back flat. Keep the arms relaxed. Do not overdo this one as you can develop soreness in your back. View the movement as a spring slowly coiling and uncoiling.

Breathing: Breathe in as you ease off and breathe out when you are lifting your shoulders.

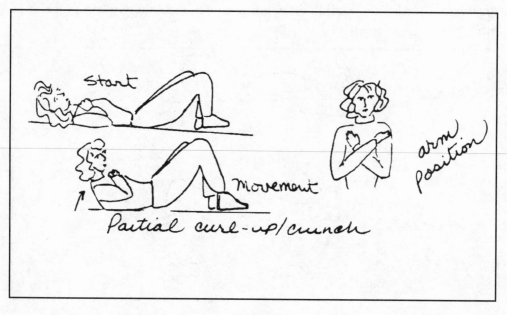

Knee to Chest:

If you do not have a disc problem, you can do this on your back, but if you do have a disc problem lie on your sides and pull your knees to your chest in accord with the following directions.

Purpose: To stretch the muscles of the lower back and to keep it stable by strengthening the back muscles.

Repetitions: Stretch once on each side.

Starting Position: Lie on your back with both legs straight out. Move the right leg so that the knee is bent and right foot is flat on the floor.

Movements:

1. Grab the right knee with both hands keeping the back flat, and gently pull the right leg towards the chest into the easy stretch for 15 seconds and then into the developmental stretch for 20 seconds. You do not have to touch the chest. Stretch the left leg out which is flat on the floor.

2. Gently ease off and slide the right leg back to the floor and slide the left leg back so that the left foot is flat on the floor and the knee is bent.

3. Gently grab your left knee with both hands and move into the easy stretch for 15 seconds and then the developmental stretch for 20 seconds. Stretch right leg out, then ease off so that left leg is flat on floor.

Final Position: On your back with both legs straight out.

Helpful Hints: Keep your back flat. Keep the head on the floor. Do not lift the straight leg off the floor. Be gentle in the stretch. Either knee should not be close to the chest.

Breathing: Exhale as you are raising your legs and holding, breathe in as you are easing off the stretch.

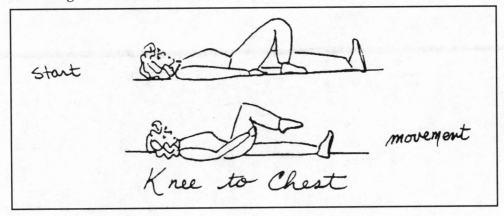

Start

movement

Knee to Chest

The Quadruped Stretch:

Purpose: Strengthening the small muscles in the back and hips.

Repetitions: Start with 3 repetitions on each side working up to 10 on each side.

Starting Position: Get down on hands and knees with knees under the hips and hands under the shoulders. Keep back straight and eyes on the floor.

Movements:

1. Raise right hand up and extend it straight out with elbow straight and palm facing down. At same time move left leg out and up behind you so that it is parallel with the floor. Hold this position for 5 seconds. Return to the starting position and repeat 9 more times.

2. Return to the starting position and then move left arm straight out with left palm facing down. At same time move right leg out behind you so that it is parallel to the floor. Hold this position for 5 seconds and return to starting position. Repeat 9 more times.

Final Position: Same as the starting position.

Helpful Hints: Do not lift hips or legs too high. Keep eyes facing down. Keep hands underneath the shoulders and knees underneath the hips.

Breathing: Breathe out while extending and breathe in when easing off the stretch.

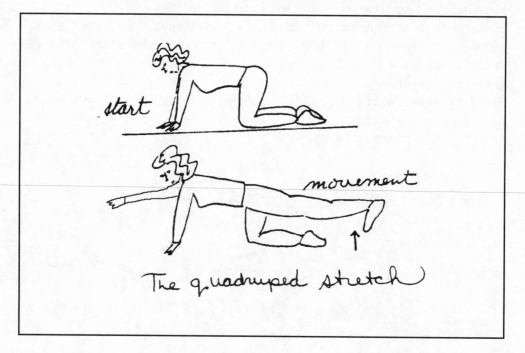

start

movement

The quadruped stretch

The Prone Extension:

Purpose: This exercise strengthens and stretches the buttock, abdominal, hamstring and back muscles.

Repetitions: 10 times on each side.

Starting Position: Lie face down on the floor with arms extended out in front of you, palms down, feet together, but toes at a 45 degree angle to the floor. The back is relaxed.

Movements:

1. Tighten the hip and abdominal muscles. Lift the left leg 6 to 8 inches off the floor, and at the same time lift the right arm, with elbow straight, 6 to 8 inches off the floor. Hold for 5 seconds. Squeeze the buttocks together at same time for 5 seconds.

2. Ease off and return to starting position.

3. Repeat on the same side 9 more times.

4. Do the opposite side by raising the right leg 6 to 8 inches off the floor and the left hand 6 to 8 inches off the floor while at the same time squeezing the buttocks together for 5 seconds.

5. Ease off.

6. Repeat the process on the same side 9 more times.

Final Position: Same as the starting position by lying on your stomach with both hands and feet extended.

Helpful Hints: Squeeze butt muscles together same amount of time arms and legs are extended.

Breathing: Breathe out when extending arms and legs and breathe in when returning to starting position.

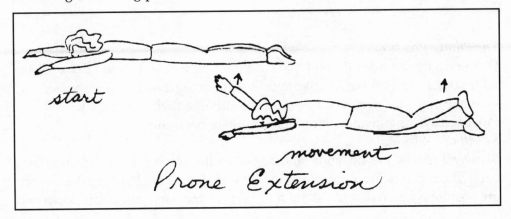

start

movement

Prone Extension

The Back Release:

Purpose: To stretch the muscles of the back and buttocks.

Repetitions: 3 times.

Starting Position: Sit upright on a chair with the feet slightly apart on the floor.

Movements:

1. View the back as a spring. Slowly curl down for a count of 5 so that the head ends up between the legs at knee level and the back of the hands are touching the floor.

2. Hold for 5 seconds.

3. Slowly curl back up to the starting position for a count of 5.

4. Repeat 2 more times.

Final Position: Sitting up straight in the chair as the starting position.

Helpful Hints: Do not bounce. Take it nice and easy. If this exercise causes a flare-up do not do it again. Curl down only to point of first resistance.

Breathing: Breathe in on the way down and exhale on the way up.

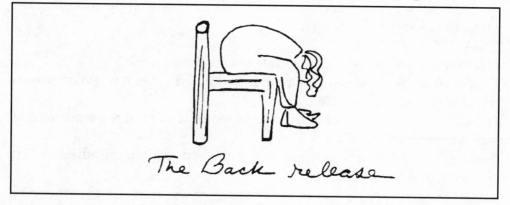

The Back release

The Elbow Press-up:

Do not do this exercise if you have facet joint problems. Discuss this exercise with your physician before attempting it. This exercise has been viewed as very effective for those who have lost the curve in their lower back.

Purpose: To maintain and strengthen the lower back curve.

Repetitions: 4 times.

Starting Position: Lie on your stomach with the forehead on the floor, legs straight out behind you with your toes at a 45 degree angle to the floor. Arms are positioned such that the shoulders are near the ears, palms flat down and the underside of the forearms on the floor. Relax all the muscles, especially those in the back and stomach.

Movements:

1. Using the forearms, press yourself up so that the bottom of your chin is about 18 to 24 inches from the floor. Keep the head foreword. Back is arched and stomach loose. Hold this position for 30 seconds.

2. Ease off, release and move back to the starting position.

3. Repeat the process 3 more times.

Final Position: Same as the starting position.

Helpful Hints: Make sure the back and stomach are sagging and loose. Do this exercise slowly and gradually and do not press too high off the floor. Keep your head straight looking forward. Do not make jerky or bouncing movements.

Breathing: Breathe in at release, exhale as press up.

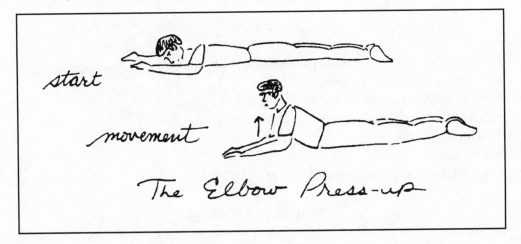

start

movement

The Elbow Press-up

The Walking Program

Walking is the most effective exercise in relieving chronic back pain. Often those with chronic back pain do not engage in significant physical activity because they fear that activity will induce more pain. Unfortunately, the opposite is generally true. Sedentary activity results in a build up of lactic acid in the muscles and allows muscles to atrophy, resulting in the weakening of the entire spinal structure, which then presses on nerves, resulting in pain. Walking, combined with the exercise program, will rebuild those muscles resulting in a stronger spinal structure and will assist in the removal of toxic lactic acid from the muscles.

The Benefits of Walking

In *Walking Through Stress, Meditation in Motion*, by Dick Harding, the benefits of walking were described as follows: " ... walking can change man's health style to normalized muscle strength, proper weight, body balance and brain equilibrium....Walking is as natural as breathing. ...daily workouts are the best brain and body relaxer anywhere on Earth." In this impressive book, the author divides walking into the following categories indicating how many calories are burned in a typical 1-hour walking session.

Type of Walking	Speed	Calories Burned
Stress Walking	1-2 mph	240 calories
Health Walking	3 mph	320
Fitness Walking	3.5 mph	440
Race Walking	5 mph	920

Equipment You Will Need

- A pair of well fitted walking shoes
- A hat, scarf, gloves and ear muffs for cold weather
- A pedometer that measures mph and distances
- Orthotics, if needed
- A watch
- A portable radio and cassette player

Breathing and Walking

In *Walking Through Stress*, the author recommends the following chi-gung breathing method:

1. Standing with your feet 12-18 inches apart, with the mouth closed, and tongue on the palate, inhale through the nose as deeply as possible, and hold the breath for 1 heartbeat. Then exhale slowly through the nose. The exhale should be as long as the inhale. Repeat this 5 times. As you gain control over the breathing, lengthen the exhalation until you can exhale for 10 seconds and then go to the next step.

2. Repeat the previous step, but in exhaling, push the breath into the abdomen, below the navel, so that little air is expelled through the nose.

3. Now integrate this with walking. Start walking slowly at first keeping with

the mouth closed at all times, inhale and exhale easily with the tongue against the palate. Take 4 steps for each inhalation and 4 steps for each exhalation. Then change after a few minutes to three steps for inhalation and 4 steps for exhalation. Then go to two steps on inhalation and 3 steps on exhalation as the walking speed is increased.

4. The final goal is two steps for each inhalation and two steps for each exhalation. The faster you walk, the faster you breathe. Keep the mouth closed with your tongue against your palate.

This walking and breathing program will lower your stress level.

What Can You Do While Walking?

Walking provides time alone when much can be accomplished. You can meditate, repeat affirmations silently or out loud, pray, plan, engage in positive self-talk, relax or listen to music or motivational tapes. As you walk, visualize that your back is getting stronger and stronger. However, walking need not be an alone time. Why not walk with friends and family? You can't beat the combination of socializing, laughter and walking. Social walking is an excellent time to tell the two jokes you have picked out for the day. Walking need not be boring; it can be invigorating and fulfilling.

A Few Tips on Walking

In *Walking Through Stress*, the author gives the following advice for health walking, which certainly applies to any form of walking:

Adopt Correct Posture:

Think straight and tall. Hold the head high, square the shoulders, and tuck in the stomach and buttocks tightly. This maximizes oxygen and blood circulation. Place your shoulders back into a T-bar shape, hold the head high and walk straight and tall.

Proper Weight Bearing and Striding:

Your weight should rest on the balls of the feet, not the heels, though you will gently touch the heels on the down step. The movement is heel and toe and heel and toe.

Relative to stride, stretch the lead leg forward as far as possible landing on the heel and then rolling it onto the ball of the foot and then shifting the body for the next step. The stride will be felt in your calf muscle. Remember the phrase "out and back" for the stride.

Arm Action:

Arms should swing and not hang, especially when health walking at 3 mph. Swinging the arms removes waste from body cells, by increasing flow of oxygen and nutrients into the blood stream. Visualize that the more you move the arms up and down, the more power, strength and healing power will come to your cells. Move the arms with fists open or closed, such that they come near your shoulder when walking briskly. Think, "push and pump" relative to arm action.

Breathing:

Use the chi gung breathing. The key words are "full and free."

Warm-up, Stretching, Cool Down, and Stretching Again:

If you are going to do a vigorous health walk at 3 mph, you need to do a mild warm up. Do some stretches, then walk, then cool down and stretch again. For a health walk, take a 5-10 minute stroll, stretch your hamstrings, thighs, trunk and groin muscles and push your arms against the wall to relieve shoulder and arm tightness. Use the stretches we have given you. After a health walk, cool down by walking more slowly for a few hundred yards and do another set of stretches.

The Walking Program

We suggest the following walking program which you need to build up to:

- 30-minute brisk morning walk-2- 2.5 mph
- 30-minute walk after lunch- 2.5 mph
- 30-minute walk after dinner-2-2.5 mph

See if this will get you up to 2 miles at your pace. If not, extend it until you hit 2 miles. If you can, extend your evening walk. Since walking is one of the best exercises for lower back pain, see if you can extend your walking and start health walking. Remember to accomplish something while you walk, either through listening to tapes, meditating, visualizing, socializing, or repeating affirmations. Try these affirmations while you walk:

Every step brings me closer to a stronger, healthier back.

Every step loosens my muscles.

Every step makes my back more comfortable.

Well, now you have the full exercise program. We recognize it is a lot of work, but it will pay off in terms of stronger and more flexible muscles and with considerable reduction in pain.

The Exercise Chart

A detailed exercise chart follows. Photocopy and use it to keep track of the daily completion of the exercise program on a weekly basis. While it is for the full workout, you can use it for the beginning workout by checking only those exercises applicable to the beginning workout.

EXERCISE LOG

Place a check in the appropriate box as exercises are completed

Week of_____

WARMUP	Repetitions (fill in)	Mon	Tues	Wed	Thur	Fri	Sat	Sun
1.Arm Circles								
2.Marching in Place								
3.Knee Circles								
4.Shaking Hands & Feet								
5.Full Body Tapping								
6.Bending Knees & Tapping								
AEROBIC								
SPECIAL STRENGTH								
1.Bent Leg Raise								
2.Straight Arm Pullovers								
3.Partial Push-Offs								
4.Partial Sit-Ups								
5.Lateral Leg Raise								
6.Rear Lateral Leg Raise								
7.Upper Back Toner								
STRENGTHENING								
1.Triceps Strengthener								
2.Pectoral Strengthener								
3.Shoulder Strengthener								
4.Shoulder & Forearm								
5.Biceps Stregthener								
6.Leg & Hip Strengtheners								
STRETCHING								
1.Calf Stretch								
2.Quadricep Stretch								
3.Standing Side Stretch								
4.Hip Flexor Stretch.								
5.Upper & Mid Back Stretch								
6.Hip Rotator Stretch								
7.Hamstring Stretch								
BACK EXERCISES								
1.Pelvic Tilt								
2.Crunches								
3.Knee To Chest								
4.Quadruped								
5.Prone Extension								
6. Back Release								
7.Elbow Pressup								
WALKING								
SOMATICS								
FELDENKRAIS								
YOGA								

CHAPTER 17

FELDENKRAIS MOVEMENT THERAPY

What Is It?

FELDENKRAIS, A MOVEMENT THERAPY, was developed by Moshe Feldenkrais, an Israeli physicist, who hurt his knees in his early thirties.

Why Does It Work?

The method re-teaches correct movement, with a minimum of effort and maximum efficiency--not through strength, but through awareness of how the body works.

Unfortunately, we barely notice that our freedom of movement and posture have been compromised by stress. Typically the strain and stresses of living manifest themselves in muscle tension resulting in low back pain. As we age, we limit our movements and do not use the full range of our muscles and joints, and they become stiff and arthritic. Feldenkrais instructs how to overcome these limitations, reconnects you with the natural ability to move and assists in regaining a full range of movement. Flexibility and coordination result from consistent use of Feldenkrais movements.

Feldenkrais is highly effective in relieving chronic back pain. It is non-stressful and the movements are easy. The daily maintenance routine featured in this chapter was provided by Feldenkrais practitioner Andrew Wright and is specifically for those with back pain. If you live in the San Francisco Bay Area, Andrew can be contacted at (415) 339-8333. To find a Feldenkrais practitioner in your area, or for books, tapes, or videos on Feldenkrais, contact:

> The Feldenkrais Guild
> 524 Ellsworth St.
> PO Box 489
> Albany, OR 97421-0143
> 1 (800) 775-2118

How Do You Do It?

Each Feldenkrais movement will be broken down into parts, with specific practice areas, until you build up to the full movement. Audio taping the practice movements in the steps noted may be a helpful idea so you do not have to refer back to the book.

Remember these important tips while learning and practicing Feldenkrais.
• Feldenkrais is 90% mental and 10% physical.
• Always be aware of the body and how the muscles and bones of each part of the body interrelate.
• Only do what is comfortable. Listen to the body. Every exercise might not be right.
• Let the exercises happen and let the body follow its natural movement.
• Use parts of the body to support each other.
• Follow the instructions carefully.
• Do not strain to reach a point; just let the body move there naturally.
• Do the movements slowly and in rhythm. Start out slowly by doing less than the stated number of repetitions.
• Since everything is interrelated, be aware of where the body is and what happens with the body in each movement.

The Feldenkrais Movement Therapy

The Whole Body Stretcher:
Purpose: To lengthen body and loosen back.
Repetitions: 15 on left side, 12 on right side.
Starting Position: Flat on back with all muscles relaxed.
Movements:
1. Gently roll onto left side with left ear on the floor, left arm and hand in front of you and right hand on hip. Legs are straight with right leg on top of left.
2. Take right hand, move it to forehead and then reach around in front and grab the head just above the left ear.
3. Gently pull head about 6-8 inches off the floor and gently return the head to the floor. Gently and slowly repeat the movement 14 more times.
4. Remove right hand from head, place it by right side and gently roll onto back. One side of the back will feel very loose. Now roll onto right side, with left hand on the outer hip, the right part of head on the floor and grasp head just above right ear with the left hand.

5. Gently pick up head with left hand, raise it 6-8 inches and return it to the floor. Repeat this movement 11 more times.

6. Return to the starting position.

Final Position: Flat on the back.

Helpful Hints:

Make the movements slow and natural; do not jerk the head or neck when moving up. Imagine how relaxed the back is becoming.

Breathing: Breathe naturally, though breathe in when lowering head and breathe out when lifting the head.

Result: Get up and walk around for a few minutes. Most of the tension should have been removed from the back.

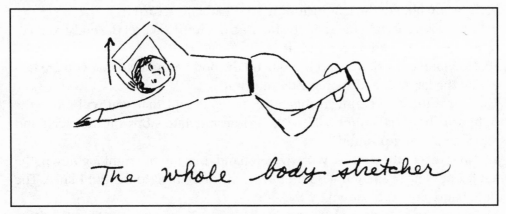

The whole body-stretcher

The Back Loosener:

Purpose: To loosen all the muscles in the back and bring you more into alignment.

Repetitions: 5 full rolling movements each on the left and right sides.

Starting Position: Flat on back, with the left and right legs straight out. Both arms are by the sides, the palms down.

Movements:

1. Imagine that the body is a clock with the feet being the 6:00, the head 12: 00, and the right side perpendicular to the right hip 9: 00 and the left side perpendicular to the left hip 3: 00.

2. Roll the right leg inwards and outwards with the leg straight 3 times. Now roll the left leg inward and outward 3 times. Now roll both legs simultaneously inwards and outwards. Sense what is happening in the hip joints.

3. Leave left leg stable but roll right leg outwards so the knee bends and then

drag the right foot along the ground so that the knee is up in the air next to left knee and the right foot is flat against the floor.

4. Slowly move the right hand only out to 9:00 and return it. Keep the right hand on the floor.

5. Now move the right hand out to 10:00 and return it. If the hand feels like turning naturally so that the palm is facing up, let it.

6. Now move the right hand to 11:00 and return it.

7. Then move the right hand to 12:00 slowly, and you will feel the body want to turn slightly to the left. Let it happen and return it. Push down on the right foot to assist you.

8. Now move the right arm out to 1:00, bending the elbow and turning the body as a whole to the left, including the head and return it.

9. Now move the right hand on the floor across until 2:00, let the body roll naturally to the left and then return it

10. Now move the right hand to 3:00, roll the body around so that you are laying on the left side and then gently return it.

11. Repeat the above movements 5 full times except that you will move the right arm from 9:00 until 3:00 without intermediate stops on the clock and return to starting position.

12. Now repeat the process with the left hand, placing the right leg down, the left leg up, knee bent and left foot flat on the floor, next to the right knee. The right hand should be down by the side.

13. Progressively move the left hand to 3:00, then 2:00, and then 12:00 on the clock.

14. When you get the left hand to 2:00 on the clock, start turning the body. Use the left foot to assist by pushing on the ground.

15. Move to 9:00 on the clock with left hand, rolling the body to the right, pushing on the left foot to assist you. Repeat this movement 5 full times except that you will not make intermediate stops on the clock and return to starting position.

Final Position: You will be lying on the back with the left leg up and left foot on floor next to right knee with right foot straight out.

Helpful Hints: Let the body flow naturally. Let the hand move naturally and if the palm wants to turn up let it turn. Make the movements very gentle and fluid; no jerking movements.

Breathing: Breathe in as you return and breathe out when you are moving into the movement.

Result: Roll up and walk around for a few minutes. All tension should be removed from the back.

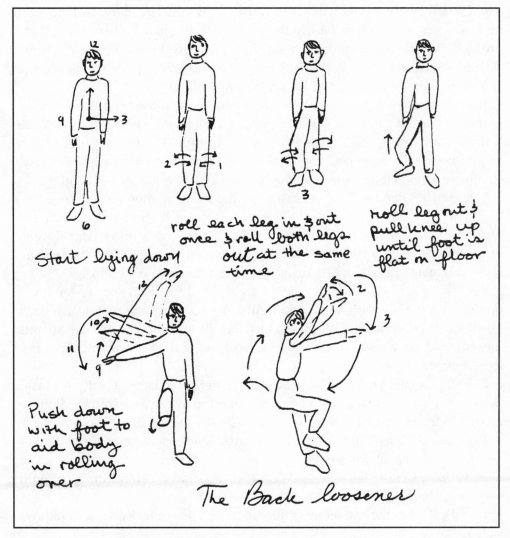

Start lying down

roll each leg in & out
once & roll both legs
out at the same
time

roll leg out &
pull knee up
until foot is
flat on floor

Push down
with foot to
aid body
in rolling
over

The Back loosener

Knee To Chest-Feldenkrais Style:
Purpose: To loosen and strengthen the muscles of the low back.
Repetitions: 3 times each for each knee to chest pull.
Starting Position: Lying on back with knees bent up, both feet on the floor, near the buttocks.

Movements:

1. Place the left hand behind the head and the right hand on the right knee cap. The left elbow is flat on the floor. Gently move the left elbow and the right knee towards each other, raising the head with the hand. Then move them away. Repeat this movement 2 more times. Be sure to rest the head on the floor after each movement. *Knee and elbow need not touch; just move into the area of comfort.* Note how the lower back rests on the floor.

2. Now reverse the process, with the right hand behind the head, the left hand grabbing the left knee cap. Gently move the right elbow and the left knee towards each other, raising the head with the right hand. Then move them away. Repeat this movement 2 more times. Rest the head after each movement. Again, knee and elbow need not touch; just move into the area of comfort.

3. Place the left hand behind the head and the right hand on the left knee cap. Gently move the left elbow and left knee towards each other, raising the head with the left hand. Then move them away. Repeat this movement 2 more times. Be sure to rest the head and elbow on the floor after each movement. Knee and elbow need not touch, just move into the area of comfort.

4. Reverse the process. Place the right hand behind the head and the left hand on the right knee. Gently move the right knee and right elbow towards each other, raising the head with the right hand. Then move away. Repeat this movement 2 more times. Be sure to rest the head and elbow on the floor after each movement.

5. Place both hands behind the head with fingers interlaced. Gently lift head from the ground, towards the knees, pressing the lower back into the floor to assist. On the return, arch the lower back slightly as you bring the head back to the ground. Raise the head about 6 inches. Do the movements slowly and rhythmically. Repeat 2 more times.

Final Position: On the back, with both hands interlaced behind the head with both knees bent, elbows and feet flat on the floor.

Helpful Hints: Do the movements slowly and in rhythm. Knees and elbows should not touch.

Breathing: Breathe out as you are lifting the head up and moving elbows towards knees, and breathe in when you are returning. After each movement, make sure the elbows are flat on the ground.

Result: Roll over and rise up and walk around. Notice how loose the back is.

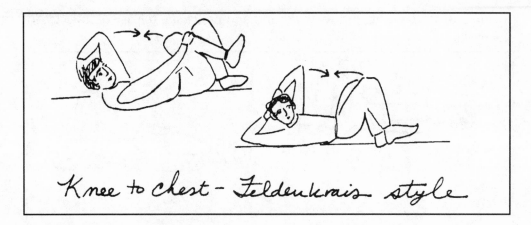

Knee to chest - Feldenkrais style

The Rolling and Lifting Pelvis:

Purpose: To loosen the back muscles and spine.

Repetitions: Roll pelvis 3 times each side raising pelvis 2 times.

Starting Position: Lying on back with both knees bent, feet near the butt and both feet flat on the floor.

Movements:

1. Press right foot into the ground and let the pelvis roll to the left side and return. Repeat 2 more times.

2. Then press left foot into the ground and let the pelvis roll to the right and return. Repeat 2 more times.

3. Notice how the spine responds and envision it as chain with the vertebrae as links in the chain.

4. Now come to rest.

5. Press both feet into the ground and begin to lift the spine off the ground, starting with the tail bone, then the sacrum, then the lower and upper part of the pelvis. Lift the spine one vertebrae at a time, with the weight of the spine hanging down. Only lift as high as is comfortable. Set the spine down one vertebrae at a time, until the pelvis is flat on the floor. Repeat the movement one more time. As you do this movement the chin moves towards the throat.

Final Position: You end with knees bent, feet flat on the floor.

Helpful Hints: Only roll the pelvis and raise the spine to a level that is comfortable. Make the rolling movements very smooth.

Breathing: Breath out as you roll to right or left and as you raise the spine, and breathe in as you return from rolling and lowering spine to the floor.

Result: Slowly stand up and walk around and notice the release of muscles in the back.

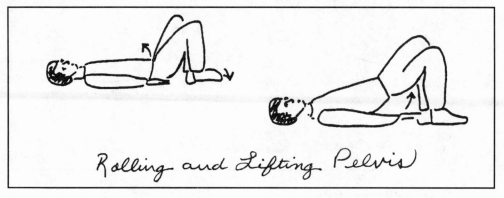

Rolling and Lifting Pelvis

The Back and Pelvic Roll:

Please note: This exercise is somewhat challenging. Wait to do it until after you have been following the exercise program for a number of weeks.

Purpose: To massage the lower back and make the legs more flexible.

Repetitions: 5 on each side.

Starting Position: Lie on the back with the knees bent and feet on the floor near the buttocks.

Movements:

1. Grab the right ankle with the right hand and left ankle with the left hand. If you can't reach that far, grab the shin bones with those hands. The arms go in between the knees.

2. Roll to the left and extend the right leg towards the ceiling, roll back towards the middle dropping the right leg and as you roll towards the right, raise the left leg towards the ceiling. In these rolls the knees are slightly bent.

3. Roll back and forth so that you roll a total of 5 times on each side, lifting the legs in the sequence noted above.

4. The movement is coming from the back and each leg is straightening out the arm.

5. Roll to the middle and release the hands from the ankles or shins.

Final Position: You are lying on the back with knees bent and feet flat.

Helpful Hints: Roll gently and not too far.

Breathing: Breathe out while exerting effort on the roll in and breathe in when rolling back.

Result: Notice how much looser the back muscles are.

174

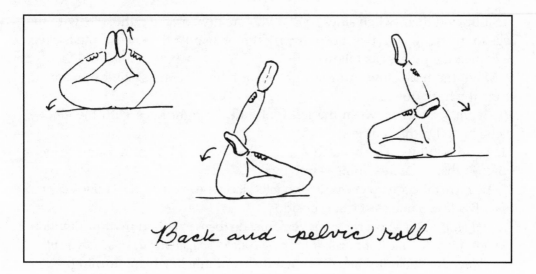

Back and pelvic roll

The Head to Knee Rock and Roll:

Please note: This exercise is somewhat challenging. Wait to do it until after you have been following the exercise program for a few weeks.

Purpose: To loosen the neck, trunk and back.

Repetitions: 4 full movements on each side.

Starting Position: On back with the knees bent.

Movements:

1. Roll to left side and sit up.

2. Position yourself so that the legs are bent to the left, with both knees pointing to the left, with the sole of the left foot resting on the right knee. The bottoms of the left and right thighs are flat on the floor. Hands are resting palms down on the floor spread out so that they are under each shoulder.

3. Begin to bend down the head to the left knee, bring head up, then bend head down again, but keep head down this time.

4. With the head down, begin to sway the whole body to the left and then to the right aiming first towards the left knee and then towards the right foot. Do this swaying motion a total of 3 times.

5. Now begin to move the head in a full circle. Circle the head up and down, first two times in a clockwise direction, then two times counter-clockwise.

6. In this movement, the whole of the spine is involved and the movement is not restricted to the neck.

7. Sit up and then switch sides so that you are now on the right side, with the legs to the right, with the sole of the right foot against the knee of the left leg.

8. Repeat the process as follows.

9. Move the head down to the right knee twice. At the second movement, leave the head down.

10. Begin to sway between the left foot and the right knee with the elbows being bent. Do this 3 times.

11. Begin to fully circle the head 2 times clockwise and 2 times counter-clockwise, so that the entire spine is moving.

12. After two full circles clockwise and counter clockwise return to the starting position.

Final Position: Same as starting position.

Helpful Hints: Make no jerking movements; do them in a fluid rhythmic motion. Do not move too far if it hurts. *If twisting bothers you, do not do this movement.*

Breathing: Breathe out when exerting effort and inhale when returning.

Result: Stand up, walk around and notice how loose the back is.

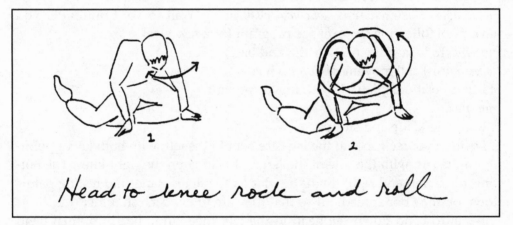

Head to knee rock and roll

The following books are highly recommended by those therapists who practice Feldenkrais therapy.

Awareness through Movement by Moshe Feldenkrais

Mindful Spontaneity by Ruth Alon, contains theory and lessons.

Relaxercise by David and Kaethe Zemach-Bersin and Mark Reese—contains simple to follow Feldenkrais routines.

(The above movements will be combined into an approximate 10 minute Feldenkrais workout. See Appendix E for the track of the CD to use with this chapter.)

CHAPTER 18

SOMATICS: LEARNING TO TAKE CONSCIOUS CONTROL OF TIGHT MUSCLES

What Is It?

SOMATICS, AN OUTGROWTH OF FELDENKRAIS, is a movement therapy developed by Thomas Hanna. Like Feldenkrais, it teaches body awareness and how our bodies move and work, and, through various exercises, to move more naturally. It is highly effective in controlling back pain.

Why Does It Work?

When under frequent stress, muscles may be chronically tight, and may become so used to being tight it may be very difficult to loosen them even when a stressful situation has passed. Soon the muscles may forget how to uncontract. Somatics re-educates the muscles.

One of the most common causes of low back pain is chronic muscle tension, the continuous contracting of various muscles in and around the back. Often after activity, the chronically-contracted muscles may not go back to their fully relaxed state right away. Thus, the muscles never rest fully. After further activity, more contraction and tightness may result, and again, the muscles may not fully relax. Unfortunately, chronically-contracted muscles do not flush out built-up lactic acid, causing soreness. The goal of Somatics is to teach full *voluntary* control over a muscle so that you can contract the muscle, relax it completely, and then rest it. Pain relief may be as simple as uncontracting the muscles and learning to move properly to avoid further tightness.

How Do You Do It?

Somatics requires mindfulness—that is, being fully present in mind and body when doing the exercises. You cannot just "go through the motions." You must practice each movement with utmost attention, being aware of the entire body. After being in chronic pain for some time, you may have learned to tune out the painful parts of the body. Thus, you may be very good at not being aware of how the body moves. Follow the guidelines below to increase body awareness and ensure an effective workout:

• Comfortable clothing will allow easy, free movement. It should be appropriate to the temperature in which you are working—that is, not chilly or too warm.

• Do the routine at a time when you know you will not be disturbed or distracted.

• Do the routine when there is enough time to do it the way it is meant to be done: mindfully, slowly, smoothly.

• Do the exercises on a soft, comfortable surface for ease of movement.

• Remember to *breathe* deeply because this keeps you in touch with the body.

• Do the exercises slowly, *mindfully*, focusing awareness on the body part(s) involved in the movements.

• Do not jerk or bounce when doing the exercises. Do them *smoothly*.

• Maintain a positive frame of mind. Hold in the mind a picture of a healthy body moving easily and smoothly the way nature intended it to.

• Above all, as with other activities in this book, be *patient*.

• Only move as far as is comfortable. Never force the movements.

The Exercises

The authors are deeply indebted to Somatics Educator Julie Rogers, who furnished the following Somatics exercise routine. She is the founder and program director of Back Strategies, a San Francisco-based back care clinic. Further information can be obtained by calling Julie Rogers at (415) 552-8990.

For practitioner referrals, books and audio and video tapes contact:

Somatics Educational Resources
1516 Grant Ave. Suite 220
Novato, CA 94945

The routine below is part of the maintenance routine of the Somatics program, designed to be used after completing the full Somatics routine noted in Hanna's book, *Somatics*, or after sessions with a Somatics educator. The routine is called the "daily cat stretch." We urge you to purchase the Hanna book and tape record the full exercise program as an adjunct to our program.

After doing the brief warm-up routine detailed in Chapter 16, perform the following "cat stretch" routine upon awakening and before bed. Each session should take about ten minutes. Mindfulness is essential because you must visualize each muscle as it contracts and relaxes while performing the movements.

Study the illustrations that follow the instructions for each part of the routine as you read the written instructions. Step-by-step movements for each part of the routine are presented, as are directions as to where in the body to focus awareness.

Arch and Flatten:

Repetitions: 5 times over a period of 30 seconds.
Starting Position: Lying on back, knees up, soles of feet on the floor. Place hands on hips.
Movements:
1. As you inhale, arch back, shifting weight to tailbone. At the same time relax the stomach muscles allowing the stomach to push up as after a big meal. Do not use the leg muscles and buttocks to accomplish the shifting of the pelvis.
2. As you exhale, shift the pelvis and lower back to the floor.
Awareness Focus: On pelvis, abdominal, and lower back muscles. When arching, concentrate on consciously contracting the muscles of the lower spine. Note the hardness of the floor pressed against the lower back. Sense that you are using the lower back muscles to accomplish the arch. Notice the stomach muscles doing the work.

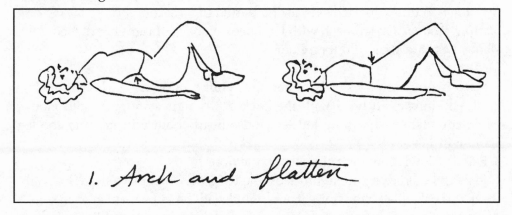

1. Arch and flatten

Arch and Flatten With Head Lift:

Repetitions: 5 times over 30 seconds.
Starting Position: Lying on back, knees up, soles of feet on floor, hands interlaced behind the head.

Movements:
1. Arch the back as you inhale, and then gently arch the neck allowing the chin to move towards the ceiling.
2. Exhale pushing lower pelvis into the floor, allowing the chin to move towards the chest with the elbows meeting in front of the face. Head and shoulders curl up off the floor, only as far as is comfortable.
Awareness Focus: On the contracted neck and lower back muscles.

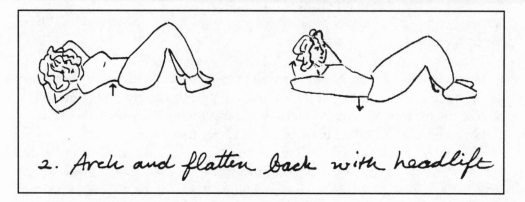

2. Arch and flatten back with headlift

On Stomach: Head, Hand and Elbow and Leg Lift:
Repetitions: 3 times on each side over a period of 30 seconds.
Starting Position: On stomach with left cheek on back of right hand, facing the elbow. Legs are straight out on floor.
Movements:
1. Perform exercise very slowly, adhering to your comfort zone when lifting leg.
2. As you inhale, lift head with the back of the right hand, arm and elbow, while simultaneously lifting left leg. Raise head about 5 inches and the leg about 6 inches.
3. Exhale, slowly lowering stomach to the floor.
4. Repeat the process 2 more times on the left side. Then place head and right cheek on back of left hand, raise it and right leg in the same manner as in step 2.
Awareness Focus: Sense the muscles surrounding the upper, middle and lower spine contract. Envision a diagonal line from right shoulder to left buttock. As you lower, feel the flow and allow yourself to sink in, noticing how the muscles relax and lengthen.

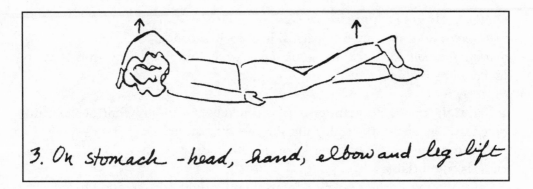

3. On stomach -head, hand, elbow and leg lift

On Back: Head, Elbow to Opposite Knee:

Repetitions: 4 times on each side in a period of 60 seconds.

Starting Position: Same as in exercises 1 and 2, on back with bent knees. Place right hand behind head and left hand near left knee.

Movements:

1. As you inhale, arch back.

2. As you exhale, flatten back to the floor, and curl the right elbow towards the left knee, with left knee moving towards right elbow. You do *not* have to touch the elbow and knee. Only go as far as is comfortable.

3. Slowly return to the floor and repeat 3 more times in a period of 60 seconds.

4. Repeat a total of 4 times on 60 seconds, on the other side, with left elbow moving towards right knee in 60 seconds.

Awareness Focus: This exercise lengthens the obliques (the muscles at the sides of abdomen and waist) and increases flexibility in the low back area. Focus on this area and imagine the muscles lengthening and increasing their flexibility.

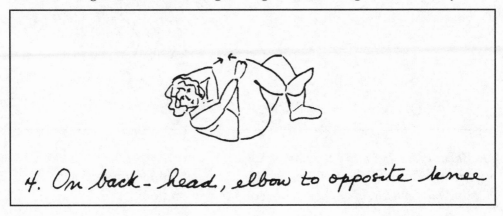

4. On back - head, elbow to opposite knee

On Back: Dishrag Spinal Twist:

Repetitions: Repeat 6 times on each side over 30 seconds
Starting Position: On back, knees up, soles of feet on floor, arms outstretched on floor at shoulder level.
Movements:
1. Roll right arm, with palm up, as far down as it will go, while at the same time turning head to the right, and roll the left arm up.
2. At same time, while holding knees together, drop them to the left, only as far as is comfortable.
3. Return to the starting position by rolling the right arm up and the left arm down, until both are outstretched.
4. Switch sides, so you are rolling the left arm down, palm up, right arm up, while at the same time turning head to the left, and then move knees to the right and return.
5. Repeat the roll and twist 5 more times on each side.
Awareness Focus: On internal and external hip muscles, or rotators. This exercise should help address sciatic pain. Flexibility will improve as you repeat this exercise.

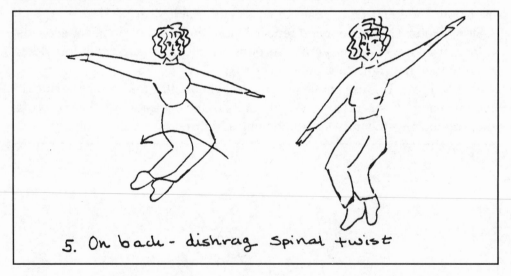

5. On back - dishrag spinal twist

On Back: Inversion and Eversion of Legs:

Repetitions: Holding position for 5 seconds, repeat 5 times on each side.
Starting Position: On back, knees up, soles of feet on floor.

Movements:

1. As you lower right knee to the floor, twist the sole of right foot as far as possible towards the ceiling, as if you were scooping ice cream with the foot. Hold the position for 5 seconds.

2. Straighten the leg.

3. Bring the leg back up and let the knee fall inwards to the left leg. Hold for 5 seconds.

4. Repeat 4 more times.

5. Change sides, so the exercise is performed a total of 5 times on the left side, lowering the left knee to the floor. Follow the same steps as with the right knee and leg.

Awareness Focus: When "scooping" with foot, focus on the lengthening of inner thigh and groin area. When leg falls inward, focus on the lengthening in the buttocks and outer hip.

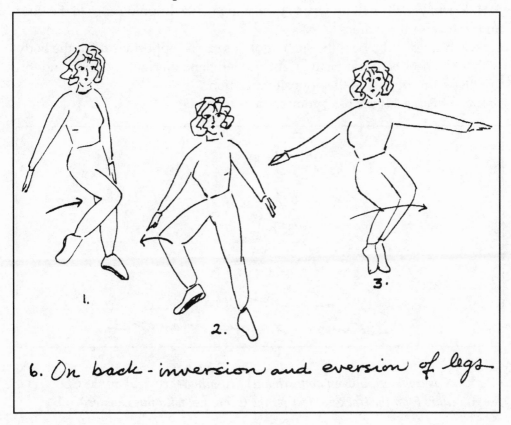

6. On back - inversion and eversion of legs

Sitting: Trunk Rotation:

Caution: This exercise is helpful for people with neck pain. However, if you have acute lower back pain, do not try this until you have practiced the rest of this routine for several weeks to increase flexibility. When you attempt this exercise, increase the range of motion *gradually.*

Repetitions: 3 times on each side of the body in a period of 60 seconds.

Starting Position: Sit with right hand on left shoulder and both knees bent facing left.

Movements:

1. Rotate trunk to the left, 3 times.

2. Hold trunk motionless at a full left turn, turn head to the right and back three times.

3. Then turn both head and trunk in alternate directions, 3 times for a full spinal twist.

4. Hold trunk to the left, lift face to the ceiling while dropping eyes to the floor and vice versa three times.

5. Switch sides and repeat the same motions on the opposite side of the body with both knees bent and facing right and left hand on right shoulder and follow steps 1 through 4 in the opposite direction.

Awareness Focus: Notice how your spine is twisting.

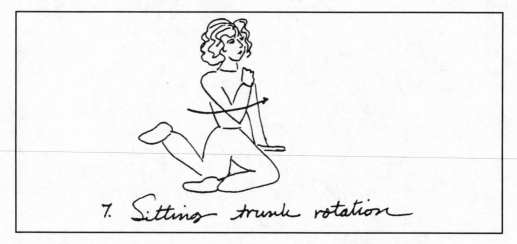

7. Sitting trunk rotation

(The above is combined into an approximately 10-minute workout on the CD. See Appendix E for the track number on the CD to use with this chapter.)

CHAPTER 19

PROPER FORM: THE CORRECT STANDING, SIT- TING, WALKING, AND LIFTING POSTURES AND HOW TO REST THE BACK FOR PAIN RELIEF

What Is It?

POSTURE relates to the position of the entire body while standing, sitting and walking.

Why Is Proper Posture Important for Back Pain Relief?

As humans, we were meant to stand erect with three natural curves (cervical, thoracic, lumbar) in our backs. For maximum functioning, we were designed to stand, walk, and sit with shoulders back, heads balanced over our spines, and our hips, trunk, knees, legs and feet in alignment. When correct posture is attained and maintained, the body is in proper alignment. Muscles are where they should be, with no unnecessary strains or pulling. When we achieve correct posture and proper alignment, pain should be significantly relieved. If the body is out of alignment, the muscles attempt to compensate for the misalignment, thereby resulting in muscle imbalances, strains, tears, and spasms.

Proper Standing Posture

Here are some suggestions to test and correct standing posture:
• Stand against a wall to test your current standing posture. The back of the head should touch the wall, there should be three natural curves in the back, and there should only be a small space between the wall and the back. If your posture deviates from these requirements, comply with the following guidelines.
• Stand tall with the chin tucked in and the ears in line with the shoulders.
• The head should not be too far forward or backward, but directly over the spine. Improper forward placement of the head can pull the rest of the body out of line and place unbalanced weight on the back.
• The shoulders should be rolled back in a comfortable position. Do not slouch or slump, as either action could increase the curves in the back, throw-

ing the body out of proper alignment.

• The pelvis should be tilted slightly forward to a position of comfort maintaining the natural curves in the back, with the stomach tucked in. If you are in pain, tilt the pelvis forward to lessen the pain. The hips should be over the heels.

• Knees should be slightly bent.

• Feet should be straight with the toes not curved excessively outward or inward.

• Distribute your weight evenly over both feet and do not stand excessively in one position.

Proper Sitting Posture

Try these suggestions to ensure correct sitting posture:

• Sit erect in a chair on the sitting bones deep in the buttocks. Let the feet and legs support the body.

• Place the feet about 10 inches apart, so that the knees are slightly over the toes and the feet are straight and flat on the floor.

• Press down on the feet, so that the weight of the body is being carried by the feet. Adjust your position and/or the chair so that this is possible. This should significantly relieve the weight on and tension in the back and reduce pain.

• Do not sit in a slumped, slouched, or other awkward position.

• To rise from the chair, press on the feet to move the body up from the chair. Do not twist or move the trunk. Move the body up to a standing position in one fluid movement.

• To sit in a chair, do not plop down in a chair. Approach the chair and position yourself so that the buttocks can gently sit on the chair. Keeping the body erect, gently sit down so that the feet will be in front, supporting your weight.

• Placing a small rolled up towel in the small of the back will assist you in not slumping forward and will help maintain the natural curve.

• Do not sit for more than 30 minutes at a time. After 30 minutes, stand up and stretch.

Proper Lifting Posture and Techniques

Improper lifting posture and techniques are often the main cause of strained backs and easily result in painful flare-ups. Use the following methods when lifting:

• Do not lift with your back. *Lift with the legs.* And bend the knees.

• Maintain proper standing posture.

• Do not lift anything excessively heavy.

• With the knees bent, move the object to be lifted close to the body, and no

higher than the chest.
- Use the thigh and lower leg muscles to lift.
- Make sure the weight is evenly distributed between the legs.
- Be careful not to twist the body.
- If you do a lot of lifting on a regular basis, purchase a back protector belt—a wrap with a suspender-like support that is placed and tightened around the lower back to stabilize it.
- Finally, get help if you think you can't lift something! Think whether you really want to risk a flare-up or additional injury.

Proper Walking

Try these tips to improve your walking:
- Start with the proper standing posture.
- Lean the body slightly forward, but not at the waist.
- Push off with the exertion in the balls of the feet.
- Do not pull the arms too far forward
- Pull the elbows back.
- Keep the back and shoulders erect and loose.
- Keep the pelvis at an appropriate level of comfort.
- Maintain chin in a level position and minimize head movement.
- Move the arms, not the whole upper body.
- Do not lock the knees.
- Land gently on the heels.
- Remain in good form for the entire duration of the walk.

In the Pain Management Contract there will be an entry entitled "proper form." It requires you to maintain proper standing, sitting, lifting, and walking postures by adhering to the above guidelines. Proper posture can go a long way in relieving back pain.

How To Rest the Back

There are four excellent positions that will rest the back and relieve pain. Try each and then use the ones that are most effective:

Yoga Corpse Pose: Lie down on the back with the head resting on the floor, arms outstretched about 6 inches from the body, with palms open, and the feet spread apart about 10 inches. Breathe deeply, using the technique for abdominal breathing presented in Chapter 7, and remain in this position for about 10 minutes. Tension will leave the back as it melts into the floor.

Press Backs: While standing in a comfortable position, place the hands on both sides of the spine in the low back area. Bend backward only to a level of comfort and hold the position for about 45 seconds to a minute. This should provide significant relief if the pain is from sitting slumped over.

The Back Stretcher: While sitting in a chair with the hands wrapped around the knees, lean forward in the chair and aim to place the head over the knees. Lean to the point of only mild resistance. Hold this position for a minimum of 2 and a maximum of 5 minutes. Come up out of the position slowly.

The Ultimate Back Relaxer: Lie on the back and scoot the buttocks towards a chair. Place the legs on the seat of the chair so that the calf muscles are fully supported by the seat. Hold this position for 15 minutes and engage in deep abdominal breathing. Visualize any pain or stiffness melting away.

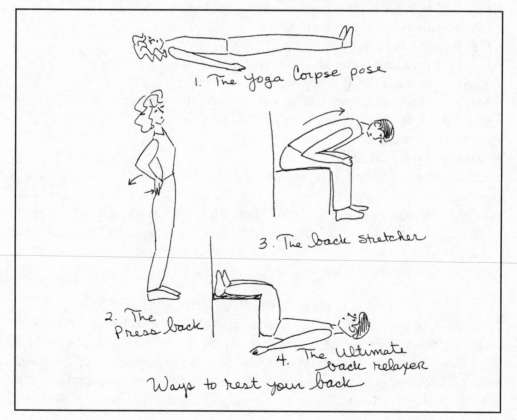

1. The yoga Corpse pose

3. The back Stretcher

2. The Press back

4. The Ultimate back relaxer

Ways to rest your back

CHAPTER 20

YOGA AND TAI CHI: ANCIENT METHODS FOR RELAXATION AND PAIN RELIEF

What are They?

BOTH YOGA AND TAI CHI are ancient practices that seek to unblock the life force energy called chi. Yoga, a Hindu practice, helps balance the energy centers of the body through various stretching and breathing exercises. Certain yoga stretches have been found to be very beneficial to back pain sufferers. Tai Chi, a Chinese martial art, is simply moving meditation. Like sitting meditation and yoga, it can be useful in a pain-control program. Both yoga and Tai Chi are for the back pain sufferer who is up and around, not for the person who is still very restricted by pain and stiffness.

Many people probably have a picture of someone twisted up like a pretzel when thinking of yoga, but many of the stretches are very simple and very effective. Through various stretches, postures, and breathing patterns, yoga promotes the smooth, even flow of energy through the body. The exercises either increase flow to places where energy is needed or release excess energy from places where it is accumulated or blocked.

In *Tai Chi: Ten Minutes to Health*, Tai Chi is described as a "series of continuous, slow, smooth, and graceful moves executed with suppleness in a relaxed manner." Though it is an ancient martial art, it is termed a "soft" martial art, and looks more like dancing. It combines breathing with its slow rhythmic movements to strengthen the body, making it more supple and flexible. It promotes inner strength, while fostering outer suppleness and softness. In China, Taiwan, and many other Chinese communities around the world, you can see people of all ages performing the gentle art of Tai Chi in parks early in the morning to start their day with a calm mind and refreshed, supple body. Volumes have been written on Tai Chi and we do not have the space here to describe all its moves completely. Most Tai Chi students learn the moves from a teacher, and then practice at home.

Although the moves for yoga and Tai Chi are generally gentle, before starting either, check with your physician or physical therapist to make sure the movements and poses are safe for your particular condition.

Why Do They Work?

Yoga breathing and postures help open up energy centers in the body (*chakras*) and regulate the flow of energy through those centers. The spine connects through nerves to the entire body and all the organs. Thus, the health of the spine relates to and affects the well-being of the whole body. Often with back pain and stiffness, you may favor the painful area, holding the body stiffly or awkwardly; this in turn creates imbalance and more stiffness in compensating areas. Yoga can help you get in touch with the body to find and correct the imbalances. Yoga is also both physically and mentally relaxing. It promotes peace of mind, patience, and discipline, all of which are useful in a pain management program.

The *chi* in Tai Chi, is the Chinese word for the life force that flows through all living things. When this force is impeded, illness may result. Tai Chi movements can help unblock energy centers, allowing smooth flow of *chi* through the body, promoting well-being. As an exercise, it works for people of all ages because it is gentle, stimulates blood circulation, loosens stiff joints, and strengthens muscles. It focuses on correct posture, and relaxing and balancing the entire body so that it can return to a natural, easy posture in which the spine is aligned properly.

Tai Chi will enhance a pain management program in several ways. It fosters mental relaxation. It relieves rather than creates stress because it does not promote frustration in the way perhaps a game of golf or tennis can, when you're not playing well. It is *moving* meditation. For those who have trouble remaining still long enough for sitting meditation, Tai Chi may be the answer. Tai Chi, like sitting meditation and yoga, fosters patience, discipline, and a calm mind—all good attributes to incorporate into a pain management program. It requires no special equipment other than soft, comfortable shoes (or bare feet if indoors) and loose clothing. It can be done in a relatively small space (about 15 square yards is adequate), indoors or out, weather permitting, and requires as little as 10 minutes a day to practice, once the moves have been mastered.

How Do You Do Them?

Yoga

If you are considerably restricted by back pain, do *not* attempt any of the yoga poses presented here, except for the "corpse" pose. We are grateful to Ambe Ray, a certified Yoga therapist, who lives in the San Francisco Bay Area, for providing this gentle Yoga routine designed to relieve back pain. Ambe Ray can be contacted at (415) 387-6975.

General Guidelines

These guidelines apply to the exercise postures in the following yoga routine.
• Study and follow the instructions and illustrations carefully.
• Do not force any moves. Be extremely gentle.
• Do not do any posture that increases pain.
• Start slowly by only doing the posture 70% of the way, gradually building up to the full posture.
• If you need pillows or chairs as supports to do the postures, use them.
• Concentrate deeply on each posture, removing all else from the mind.
• Do the movements slowly and smoothly. Do not jerk or bounce.
• Try to achieve the final position in about 8 to 12 seconds.
• Hold the position about 10 seconds, though beginners should hold it for no more than 4-5 seconds. Work up to 10 seconds gradually.
• Repeat the exercises 2 to 4 times, depending on comfort level.
• Rest between postures.
• Breathe *out* when exerting effort, breathe *in* at other times.
• Do not skip the corpse pose, requiring 10 minutes of total relaxation at the end of the entire yoga routine. This is vital to a successful yoga routine.
• Do the warm-up routine in Chapter 16, before commencing the Yoga routine.
• Enhance the Yoga session by closing the eyes while doing the postures. Burn incense and listen to soothing music.

The Yoga Postures and Stretches

Knee To Chest With Extended Leg:
Starting Position: On back, legs out straight on floor, with arms by sides.
Movements:

1. Slowly raise the right leg towards chest, while putting hands around the right knee. Pull the knee in towards chest as far as is comfortable.
2. Extend left leg out at the same time to achieve a mild stretch.
3. Hold the position.
4. Gently return to the starting position.
5. Repeat the same movements pulling the left leg towards the chest and extending and stretching the right leg.
6. Finish in starting position.

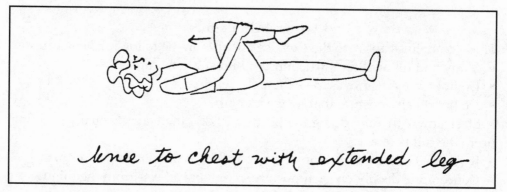

knee to chest with extended leg

Circling of Knees:

Starting Position: Lying on the floor with knees bent up and feet near the buttocks.
Movements:

1. Place hands on the knees and gently draw them towards chest to a position of comfort.
2. Make small gentle circles by rotating the knees clockwise 3 to 5 times and reverse the process.
3. Finish in starting position.

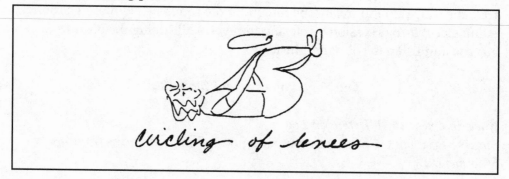

circling of knees

Double Knee to Chest:

Starting Position: Lying on your back with knees bent and feet on the floor near the buttocks.

Movements:

1. Gently place hands around both knees.
2. Gently pull the knees towards chest to a position of comfort and hold. Keep the back on the floor.
3. Return to starting position, and finish there.

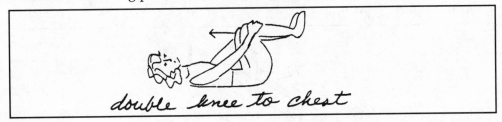

double knee to chest

Knee Drops:

Starting Position: Lie on your back, arms perpendicular to the body, knees bent and feet drawn up to buttocks.

Movements:

1. Gently drop the knees to the left to a level of comfort. They need not go all the way to the floor. At the same time turn the head to the right.
2. Return to center.
3. Gently drop knees to the right and at the same time turn the head to the left.
4. Return to center.
5. Finish in starting position.

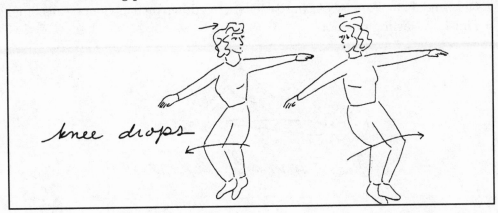

knee drops

Piriformis Stretch:

Starting Position: Lie on the floor with both knees bent up and feet near the buttocks.
Movements:

1. Move your right knee forward towards your chest.
2. Place both hands around the back of the right knee and pull it gently towards the chest.
3. Return to starting position.
4. Do the same movements with the opposite leg and return to center.
5. Finish in starting position.

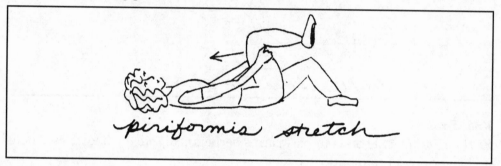

Spinal Lifts:

Starting Position: Lying on the floor with legs straight out and arms by the side.
Movements:

1. View the spine as a strand of pearls. Gently lift each vertebrae off the floor, one at a time until the spine is off the floor. Notice the gentle stretch. Do this slowly and gently.
2. Hold and then return by placing each vertebra down on the floor one at a time.
3. Finish in starting position

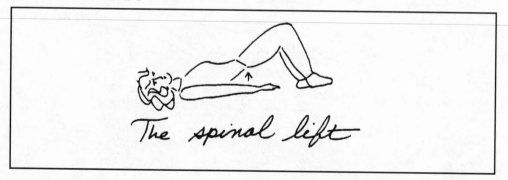

The Child's Pose:

Starting Position: Sitting on the floor.

Movements:

1. Kneel and sit back on your haunches.
2. Gently pull your head forward so that your forehead is on the floor with arms by your sides.
3. Knees should be spread with your trunk resting in between the knees.
4. After you have mastered the above, extend and stretch the arms out in front of you and move your buttocks towards the feet.
5. Return to starting position.
6. Finish in the starting position.

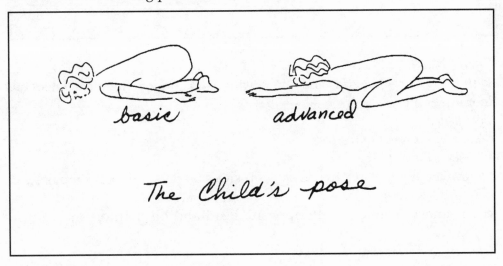

basic   *advanced*

The Child's pose

Cat Stretch:

Starting Position: Hands on floor under the shoulders, and knees on floor under the hips.

Movements:

1. Slowly begin to arch the back vertebrae by vertebrae like a cat, until you reach a comfortable arch.
2. Chin should be tucked in when this is completed.
3. Starting at the rear, lower your spine vertebrae by vertebrae, with the head finally lifting up.
4. Repeat the movement, always remember to exhale on arching and inhale on

the lowering of the spine.

5. Finish in Starting position.

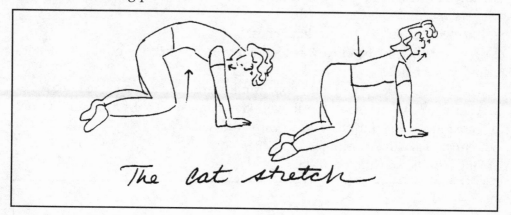

The cat stretch

Lateral Bend:

Starting Position: On hands and knees, with hands under shoulders, knees on floor under hips.

Movements:

1. Move your head to the left.
2. Look at the left hip.
3. Move left hip towards the head. Keep knees on floor and move hip only.
4. Return to center.
5. Do same movement with opposite head and hip motion and return to center.
6. Finish in the starting position.

lateral bend

Forward Bend:

Starting Position: Sitting with legs straight out on floor and arms by the sides. Place a folded pillow on your thighs for support.

Movements:

1. Bend the body over the pillows with arms outstretched towards your feet. Hold the position.
2. Slowly sit back up.
3. When you become more flexible, remove the pillow.
4. Finish in the starting position.

forward bend with cushion

The Triangle:

Starting Position: Standing with feet slightly out from shoulders and arms outstretched. Move the left foot slightly to the left.

Movements:

1. Gently bend the body to the right as far down as is comfortable grasping the right thigh or leg with right hand. Left hand is reaching for the sky.
2. Hold and then gently return to the starting position.
3. Repeat using the opposite arms, bend to the left and move the right foot slightly to the right. Return to the starting position, and finish there.

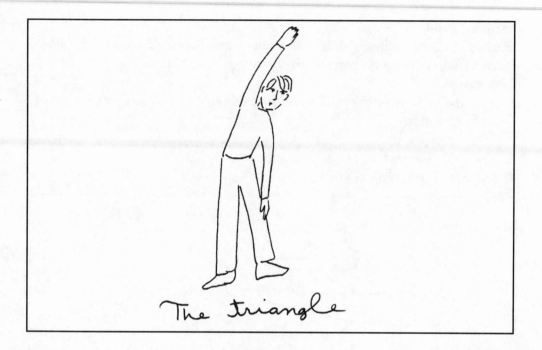

The triangle

The Corpse Pose—Total Relaxation:

Starting Position: Lying on your back with arms out to the sides and legs and feet extended out on floor.

Movements:

1. Extend arms out to about a 45-degree angle and move the feet out so they are further out than the shoulders. Turn the feet out and keep the palms open and facing up.

2. Engage in deep abdominal breathing.

3. Maintain this pose for 10 minutes.

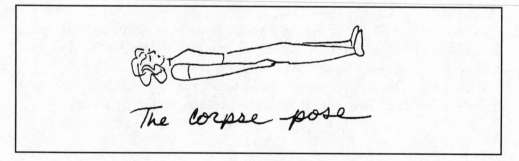

The corpse pose

Yoga Instruction

There are yoga institutes in many cities, often recreation departments and community colleges offer instruction in yoga. If you take a class, be sure to *check with your doctor first.* Also, be sure to take a class with a reputable, experienced instructor, and also talk with the instructor to make sure that he/she understands your needs and/or limitations and that the class would be right for you. It is best to stick with Hatha Yoga, the most gentle form of yoga.

Yoga Resources: Books and Video Tapes

There are many excellent yoga books on the market. We recommend two that focus on using yoga to help those with back problems:

The Yoga Back Book by Stella Weller

Back Care Basics by Dr. Mary Pullig Schatz

Video tapes are especially effective in teaching Yoga. Look for those that teach Hatha Yoga. For back pain patients, we would recommend yoga videos designed for pregnant women, as these are the most gentle of all.

(See Appendix E for the CD track to be used in conjunction with this chapter.)

Tai Chi

There are 18 or 37 basic movements (depending on which book you read) in an interlinked series consisting of gentle, often circular or pushing movements of the hands and feet, performed very slowly and mindfully while standing up. The names of the movements translated from Chinese are picturesque and even poetic: "parting the horse's mane" and "wave hands like clouds," for example. While performing the movements, the Tai Chi student also centers his/her body by focusing on a spot just below the navel, called the "tan tien," by the Chinese and believed to be the source of the body's *chi.* Some typical Tai Chi moves are illustrated below. Specific instructions are not presented as you should learn Tai Chi from an instructor or a video.

Books and Videos on Tai Chi

You will find numerous books on Tai Chi in your public library or in any major bookstore. The two titles listed below are fully illustrated.

Tai Chi: Ten Minutes to Health by Chia Siew Pang and Goh Ewe Hock

The T'ai Chi Workbook by Paul Crompton

You will find numerous videos on Tai Chi at your local library or video store.

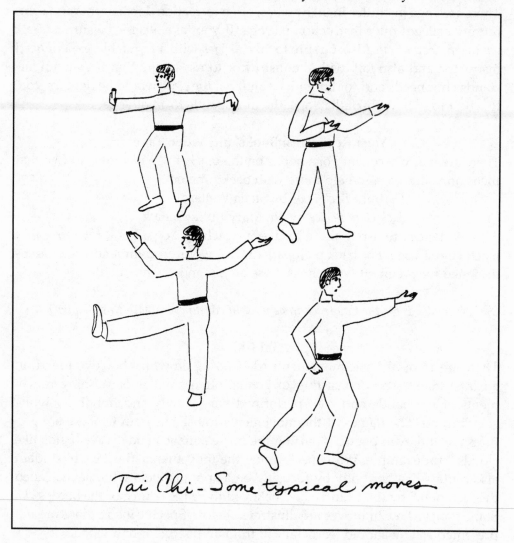

Tai Chi - Some typical moves

Some Hints Before You Start Either Yoga or Tai Chi

• Check with your physician or physical therapist.

• We suggest you read or view any Tai Chi or yoga book, video, or other instruction *all the way through* to thoroughly understand the principles before beginning.

•If you take a yoga or Tai Chi class, be sure the instructor is aware of your problems and/or special needs with regard to your back.

• It is helpful to remember that yoga and Tai Chi take some time to learn. Their value lies in their benefits to your long-term back health and to your overall well-being, rather than as immediate solutions to chronic pain.

• Only you can decide if the benefits are worth the investment of time it will take to learn. As a tool for stress and anxiety relief and creating peace of mind, both yoga and Tai Chi have definite benefits.

CHAPTER 21

ACUPRESSURE AND REFLEXOLOGY

I N REFLEXOLOGY AND ACUPRESSURE, the fingers and thumbs
are used to exert pressure on various parts of the body to relieve pain and
promote healing. The main difference between the two is in theory and
technique, but for all practical purposes they can be used together to relieve
back pain and associated anxiety and depression.

What Are They?

In reflexology pressure is applied with the fingers and thumbs to specific
points on the feet, ears, or hands. These points correspond to different parts
of the body such as the back, various muscle groups, and internal organs. The
reflexology discussion will cover only points on the hands because you can
easily and unobtrusively access these points in any setting.

Acupressure is an ancient healing technique, in which finger or thumb pressure is placed on specific points on the body. Acupressure is similar in principle to acupuncture, in which needles are inserted. The main distinction
between reflexology and acupressure is that in acupressure points *all over* the
body are activated, whereas in reflexology, these points are limited to the ears,
feet, and hands. However, in this chapter we refer to both acupressure and
reflexology points as *healing points,* and they are referred to by number on the
charts at the end of the chapter.

Why Do Acupressure and Reflexology Work?

The key to both reflexology and acupressure is the concept of chi, the vital
energy flowing throughout the body. Indeed, in Chinese medicine, practitioners seek to balance and harmonize the body to ensure an uninterrupted flow
of *chi.* This is the foundation of Chinese healing arts. *Hands on Healing,* by the
editors of *Prevention Magazine,* describes the human body as "a network of
highways and byways called meridians. These meridians weave through

every one of the body's vital organs, the bloodstream, the bones and through the muscles. Along these roads travel not cars and trucks but "chi." Illness occurs when chi is blocked in the organs or along these meridians. According to *Hands on Healing*, "with the touch of the fingers [acupressurists] can influence the flow of *chi*, and most important break up the traffic jams that can rob one of vitality and good health." Theory aside, the important thing is that acupressure and reflexology *work* and are easy to learn.

How Do You Do It?

The charts at the end of the chapter, one each of the left and right hands, front and back, and front and rear views of the body, show the location of various healing points. The general techniques and time periods to apply pressure will be discussed, and then more specifically described in the instructions for each point. While it is best to use all the points, try each out to see which ones give you the most relief, and note those down. Each healing point is noted by number on the charts. To find the healing points, apply pressure with the thumb or index finger until a dull ache or some slight tenderness or soreness is felt.

Pressure Techniques

Thumb Pressure: The thumb can exert the greatest pressure on a healing point. In general, place the thumb on the point at approximately a 45-degree angle or so that the ball of the thumb is directly over the healing point. Use the fingers to anchor the thumb by placing pressure on the area of the body or hand somewhat opposite the thumb. Use a firm rolling motion over and around the point as you massage it until you feel slight pain or an ache. Apply enough pressure so that you feel the pain, but do not make it excessively painful.

Index Finger Pressure: While the thumb is generally ideal to place pressure on the healing point, you may need to apply index finger pressure due to the location of the point. Place the index finger at an approximate 45-degree angle to the healing point and use the thumb somewhat opposite the index finger as well as the other fingers to anchor the index finger on the healing point. Use a firm rolling motion over and around the point to massage it until you feel the slight pain indicating you are activating the point. Again, do not apply excessive pressure.

Index and Middle Finger Pressure: Some healing points will require extensive massage over and around the point (generally those in the abdominal area) and will require using both index and middle finger pressure at an approximate 30-degree angle to the point, massaging in a large circular motion. Apply enough pressure to produce a slight ache. In using this form of pressure, the thumb and other fingers will not be used as an anchor point.

Pointed Objects: Some areas may be so small that pressure should be applied with a pencil's rubber eraser or an acupressure tool, or so large and diffuse that using an instrument like a plastic or metal comb will be required to activate the points.

Electrical devices: There are a number of acupressure devices on the market which send an electrical charge into the acupressure point with a plunger device on the instrument. Using this on the healing points should enhance healing point therapy. Plunge the device about 20 times for each healing point.

What You Need to Know Before You Start

How long to apply pressure: The experts vary as to how long pressure should be applied. While some say healing points should be pressured for as little as 14 seconds, others suggest one to two minutes. Experimentation for effectiveness is the key. Based on experience using the *Sound Techniques for Healing, Chronic Pain,* audio tapes authored and recorded by Dr. Robert Friedman and Kelly Howell, we recommend a period of approximately 45 seconds of pressure to activate each point. The points for anxiety relief and mood elevation may be massaged for a minute or so.

Breathing: While activating the healing points, deep abdominal breathing is necessary. Refer to Chapter 7 for breathing techniques.

Visualization: Stephanie Rick, in *The Reflexology Workout,* suggests that you visualize the area you are hoping to heal. If your muscles are tight or sore, visualize those muscles releasing, becoming less tense, or in the case of burning pain, visualize the flames dying out as you apply pressure to the healing points. Visualize the smooth, unimpeded flow of chi through the body.

The Healing Points

There have been extensive research, practice, and discussions amongst professionals on the appropriate healing points for chronic pain, anxiety, and depression. While an entire book could be devoted to this subject, from actual experience we have selected those points we believe to be the most effective. Some points were discovered by the authors through trial and error and are not reflected in the literature. Other points are very commonly known and are noted as *traditional*. First, we will describe the effective healing points for chronic pain and chronic low back pain, and then those that will relieve anxiety and nervousness, and elevate your mood. The best way to learn the points is to look at the location of the point on the chart, and read instructions for locating and activating the points.

The Healing Points for Chronic Pain and Chronic Low Back Pain

Healing Point #1:
Location: On the back of the hand, about 1 inch below the juncture at the bottom of the little and ring fingers. Use index finger to find the sore or achy point.
Technique: Press left index finger into the sore point on the back of right hand at an approximate 45-degree angle. Anchor the hand so that the thumb is touching the palm and exert pressure with finger until you feel a slight ache. Massage over and around the point for approximately 45 seconds. Massage the point on the right hand and then switch to the left hand.
Source: Traditional

Healing Point #2:
Location: On the web between thumb and index finger.
Technique: Using the left index finger and the thumb, grasp the web between the right thumb and index finger, with the index finger on the top and the thumb directly underneath it. Squeeze thumb and index finger together, massaging up and back until you locate a slight ache. Then deeply massage the point back and forth for 45 seconds. Repeat the same technique with right thumb and index finger on the left hand.
Source: Traditional

Healing Point #3:
Location: On the outer side of each thumb, from the top of the thumb progressing downward to the large wrist crease.
Technique: With the right palm facing you, reach behind it and place left thumb at an approximate 45-degree angle on the outside of the top of the right thumb, grasping the inner part of the right thumb with the remaining fingers on left hand. Apply pressure on the right thumb with the left thumb and massage down the outside of the thumb to the large wrist crease. Massage each sore point for approximately 30 seconds in a circular motion until you reach

the wrist. Repeat on the left hand with the right thumb. This area of the thumbs duplicates the lower spine.

Source: The Reflexology Workout, Rick, Pages 98-101.

Healing Point #4:

Location: With palms up, across the wrist from left to right where the wrist intersects with the bottom of the hand.

Technique: Place the left thumb at a 45-degree angle on the left side of right wrist with right palm up. Use the remaining fingers of left hand to anchor the left thumb by pressing into the back of the right wrist. Slowly, in a small circular pattern, massage across the wrist, stopping at tender points and massaging for about 15 seconds on each. Repeat the same process on left hand using right thumb. These portions of the wrist represent the sciatic nerves.

Source: The Reflexology Workout, Rick, pages 86-89.

Healing Point #5:

Location: In the middle of the fold of the knee at the back of the leg.

Technique: Using the left thumb at a 90-degree angle, locate the sore point in the middle of the fold at the back of the right knee. When that is located, use the fingers of left hand to grab onto the shin bone and then gently massage the sore point with the right thumb in a circular manner for approximately 45 seconds. Repeat the same technique on left leg using right thumb.

Source: Traditional

Healing Point #6:

Location: On left and right sides on the pelvic bones at the sore point.

Technique: Place right thumb at a 90-degree angle to the pelvic bone on right side. Applying pressure with the tip of right thumb, feel for the sore point, and then apply steady massaging pressure for at least 45 seconds. Repeat the same process with left thumb on left pelvic bone. This is an especially effective healing point when walking. Steady pressure on the sore points while you walk will reduce or eliminate pain and loosen tight muscles. Alternatively, if you cannot find any sore points, apply steady pressure with the thumb nail in these areas until pain subsides or muscles relax.

Source: Discovered by the Authors.

Healing Point #7:

Location: Approximately 3 inches below the armpit on each side of the body. When sore points are located with thumb pressure, or tight muscles loosen, you have located the point.

Technique: With right thumb at a 90-degree angle, press into the upper right side approximately 3 inches below right armpit. When you notice soreness, or muscles in the mid- or upper back begin to loosen, you have located the point. Apply steady thumb pressure for approximately 45 seconds. Repeat on the left side with the left thumb.

Source: Discovered by the Authors.

Healing Point #8:

Location: On the center of the palms of the left and right hands, below the finger pads, directly below the space between the middle and ring fingers.

Technique: Grasp the right palm with left thumb in the center of the palm, while anchoring the thumb with all four fingers of left hand directly on the back of right hand for maximum amount of left thumb pressure. Firmly massage the tender point in the center of the palm for about 45 seconds. Repeat the same process with right thumb on left palm. This point relaxes the diaphragm and solar plexus and is extremely effective. You may want to massage these points alternately three or four times.

Source: The Reflexology Workout, Rick, pages 94-97.

Healing Point #9:

Location: At the back of the right and left legs midway between the knee crease and the top of the rear portion of the ankle, at the sore point on the calf muscle.

Technique: Using left thumb, locate the sore point on the calf muscle on right leg, generally in the middle of the belly, or flat part of the muscle. Grab the right shin bone with the four fingers of the left hand and in a circular motion, massage the sore point with moderate pressure for about 45 seconds. Repeat the same process with right hand on left calf muscle.

Source: Traditional

Healing Point #10:

Location: Located in the depression directly to the rear of the large round ankle bone on the outside of both ankles.

Technique: Cross right leg over left leg and place left four fingers on the top ankle bone of the right ankle. Then with left thumb feel for the sore point in the depression behind the large round ankle bone, and apply pressure to the sore point with the left thumb, massaging over and around the sore point for about 45 seconds. Repeat the process in reverse for the healing point on the left foot.

Source: Traditional

Healing Point #11:

Location: Approximately one inch behind the split between the large and second toes on the upper part of the foot in the depression between the large and second toe bones on the achy point.

Technique: Cross right leg over left leg. Place index finger in the depression on the upper part of foot as noted above. Grab the rest of foot with the remaining fingers and thumb to anchor the index finger over the healing point. Bend the index finger so the maximum amount of pressure can be applied and massage the point in a circular motion for 45 seconds. Repeat the same process in reverse for the point on the left foot.

Source: Chronic Pain, Sound Techniques for Healing, Friedman & Howell, point #11 on the audio cassette program.

Healing Point #12:

Location: Approximately three inches up from the inside ankle bone at the sore or achy point.

Technique: Cross right leg so that it is sitting on top of the left knee. With the left thumb, feel for the sore point as noted above. Place the left fingers around the front bottom portion of the leg and ankle and bend the thumb to a 90-degree angle, on the sore point and massage in a circular motion for approximately 45 seconds. Repeat the same process in reverse for the point on left leg.

Source: Chronic Pain, Sound Techniques for Healing, Friedman & Howel, point #10 on the audio cassette

Healing Point #13:

Location: Approximately three inches below the knee caps on the sore points next to the shin bones on the inner portion of the legs.

Technique: While sitting, place both feet on the floor about 4 inches apart in front of you. Place both hands on the knee caps, move the thumbs down the inside portion of legs just below the knee caps and feel for the sore points just inside of the shin bones. Bend your thumbs so that the upper segment of your thumbs is pressing on the points at a 90-degree angle and then anchor these points simultaneously with your remaining fingers around the upper part of the shin bone. Massage the sore points in a deep circular motion simultaneously for 45 seconds.

Source: Chronic Pain, Sound Techniques for Healing, Friedman & Howell, point # 9 on the audio cassette program.

Healing Point #14:

Location: Fold your arms. This point is located about one inch up from the end of elbow crease on the outside of the arm. Locate the sore spot with your thumb.

Technique: With right arm folded across chest, place the left thumb at a 45-degree angle about one inch above the elbow crease in the right arm. Anchor the thumb by placing fingers tightly around the elbow. Massage over and around the point in a deep circular motion for about 45 seconds. Reverse the process, massaging the corresponding spot on the left arm with the right thumb.

Source: Chronic Pain, Sound Techniques for Healing, Friedman & Howell, point #3 on the audio cassette program.

Healing Point #15:

Location: At the crown of the head, the highest point on the head. Use the index and middle finger to find the sore point.

Technique: Place index and middle fingers on spot noted above, and grasp the head with thumb and remaining fingers. Use the index and middle fingers to massage over the point in a deep circular motion for about 45 seconds.

Source: Chronic Pain, Sound Techniques for Healing, Friedman & Howell, point #1 on the audio cassette program.

The Healing Points To Uplift Your Mood

Most of the healing points in this section are the *same* as those used to treat chronic pain, (Healing Points 1-15) and while the technique is basically the same, the difference is in the length of time the point is massaged. These points will be noted by their number from the foregoing section when they are the same. Please refer to the instructions under that number in the previous section and the charts at the end of the chapter.

Healing Point #8:

Location/Source: See healing point #8.

Technique: Use the same technique, but to uplift your mood, massage the point for one minute and repeat.

Healing Point #3:

Location/Source: See healing point #3.

Technique: Use the same technique, but to uplift your mood, massage the thumbs for a total of five times alternately on each thumb for a period of 30 seconds for each massage.

Healing Point #16:
Location: In the center of the thumb pad on each thumb.
Technique: Place left thumb nail down in the center of the right palm. Use the middle finger of the right hand to deeply massage the center of the left thumb pad for about 15 seconds in a circular motion until you feel a slight pain or ache. Repeat the process a total of five times. Then massage the center of the right thumb pad using the left middle finger in the same manner.
Source: The Reflexology Workout, Rick, Pages 82-85.

Healing Point #17:
Location: About $1^1/_2$ inches below the belly button.
Technique: Place the pads of the index and middle fingers of the right hand at a 45-degree angle 1 1/2 inches below the belly button. Massage this area in a deep circular motion for about one minute
Source: Depression, Sound Techniques for Healing, Friedman and Howell, point #9 on the audio cassette program.

Healing Point #15:
Location/Source: See discussion under healing point #15.
Technique: Use the same technique but massage the point for one minute.

Healing Point #14:
Location/Source and Technique: See healing point #14. Massage for about one minute.

Healing Point #13:
Location/Source and Technique: See healing point #13. Massage for about one minute.

Healing Point #12:
Location/Source and Technique: See healing point #12. Massage for about one minute.

Healing Point #18:
Location: The belly button.
Technique: Place the right index finger at a 45-degree angle in the belly button. Massage deeply in a circular motion for about one minute.
Source: Depression, Sound Techniques for Healing, Friedman and Howell, point # 10 on the audio cassette program.

When to Use the Healing Point Techniques

It is recommended that you start the day off with mood uplifter healing points. Do the workout for pain control at lunch time and again at dinner time, and end the day with the mood uplifter workout if you have time.

When you have a painful period, use those healing points in the chronic pain section that help the most. Indeed, you can easily massage those points on the hands at anytime without notice by other people. Using the healing points on a daily basis will increase their effectiveness because they not only unblock the chi, but also promote healing. It would be helpful to tape the workout with music.

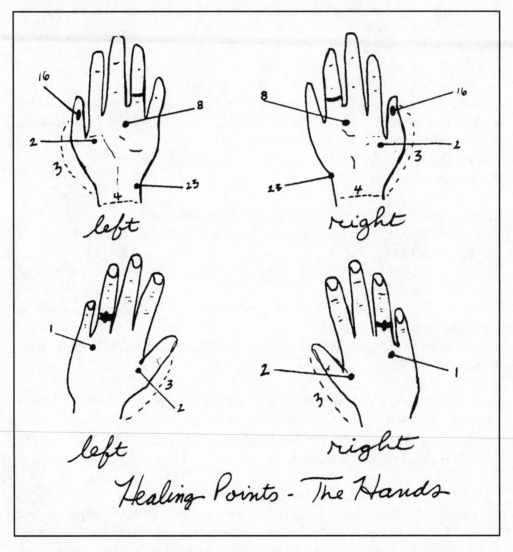

Healing Points - The Hands

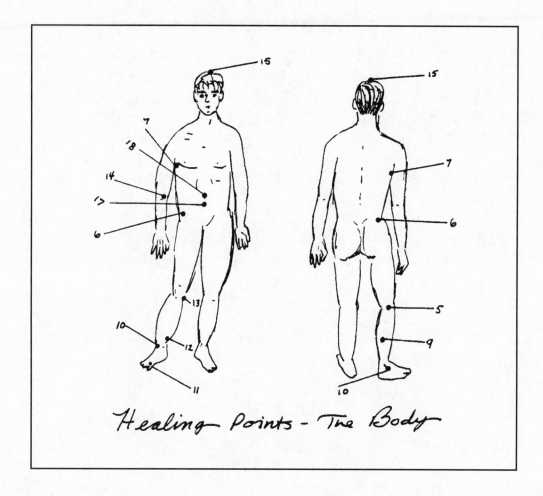

Healing Points - The Body

CHAPTER 22

OTHER FORMS OF ENERGY WORK OFFERING PAIN RELIEF

Introduction

WE DEVIATE FROM THE NORMAL CHAPTER FORMAT to present additional forms of energy work proven to be effective for back pain relief. These include: 1. Touch for Health; 2. Reiki; 3. Polarity Therapy; 4. Vibrational Healing Massage; and 5. Chi-gung. In briefly discussing each modality, we will describe the general techniques, suggest book and video references, advise how to find practitioners and whether self-help techniques are applicable.

Why is Energy Work Successful in Pain Relief?

Eastern medicine theorizes that blocked *chi* is the basic cause for most disease and pain. Energy work focuses on clearing *chi* blockages in the organs and muscles, and along the 14 meridians, or pathways, through which *chi* flows in the body. Once the blockages are cleared, the *chi* is balanced and then pain relief is normally achieved. As was explained in Chapter 21, acupressure points act like circuit breakers and once activated have the power to clear *chi* blockages. The techniques we will discuss use points on the body and various forms of touch or massage to clear chi blockages. In our opinion, and based on actual experience, effective energy work is one of the best and fastest forms of back pain relief. Generally, you need to consult a practitioner of these techniques, though each practitioner will likely offer advice on how some of the techniques can also be used at home.

ENERGY WORK MODALITIES

TOUCH FOR HEALTH

Theory and Techniques

Touch for Health is highly scientific energy work for pain relief, developed by a chiropractic doctor, John Thie. It is practiced all over the world. Blocked *chi* is identified and unblocked through muscle testing and massage of various points and meridians on the body. A Touch for Health practitioner will generally test 14 basic muscle groups to ascertain if the tested muscle is weak, out of balance, or over energized. Muscle testing consists of having the client resist about 2 pounds of pressure placed on arms or legs, depending on the muscle being tested. If the client can successfully resist the pressure, generally the muscle is in balance and no further adjustments are needed. For example, to test the lower trapezius muscle (shoulder muscle), the client is instructed to stretch his arm out perpendicular to his body. The practitioner will gently, with two pounds of pressure, attempt to pull the arm down. If the arm is moved down, that means that the muscle is underenergized and out of balance. Adjustments are needed. Both arms are tested. The practitioner will re-energize the muscle by 1. massaging identified nuero-lymphatic points on the front and back of the body; 2. massaging an associated meridian or energy pathway; 3. teaching the client how to hold various vascular points on the head; and 4. holding identified acupressure points to strengthen or weaken the muscle.

Muscle testing accesses inner intuition and can be used to identify what foods and supplements are good for you and what emotional issues are bothering you. Overall it is extremely powerful work with fast results.

References
The *Touch for Health Manual* sets forth the entire modality in great depth in an easy to understand format. It is available in bookstores.

Referrals
Contact the Institute for Kinesiology at 1(800) 501-4878 for practitioner referrals. If you live in the San Francisco Bay Area, Andrew Morris is an excellent teacher and practitioner who can be reached through the Institute.

Self Help
By working with a practitioner muscle groups that are out of balance and under energized can be identified. Once this is done, you will be instructed how to identify and massage the various neuro-lymphatic and neuro-vascular points associated with muscle imbalances. Additionally, the practitioner should be able to locate the primary meridian that will reset the body's entire

energy system if properly massaged.

There is an excellent resource book, *Self Help for Stress and Pain Relief* by Elizabeth and Hamilton Barhydt, with simple energy balancing exercises based on Touch for Health principles. The exercises, including a low back balancing technique, are highly effective. A video demonstrating the exercises is also available. The book or video can be ordered from:

> Loving Life
> 22675 Prospect Heights
> Groveland, Calif. 95321

REIKI

Theory and Techniques

Many different types of Reiki are practiced around the world. It originated in Japan and was brought to the U.S. after WWII. The "ki" in Reiki is the Japanese word for "chi." Generally the client is placed fully clothed on a massage table and the practitioner either places his/her hands above or on various points on the body for energy healing work. The practitioner allows life force energy to flow through his/her hands into the client. Depending on the Reiki system, massage and pressure on various points on the body may also be used.

References

Reiki Plus Natural Healing by David G. Jarrell
Reiki Plus Professional Practitioner's Manual by David G. Jarrell
Essential Reiki by Diane Stein

Referrals

Check the local phone book or ads in weekly alternative newspapers. Ask the Reiki practitioner for references.

Self Help

Excellent self-help routines, including those for treating the back are contained in *Reiki Plus for Natural Healing* by David G. Jarrell. There are three degrees in Reiki, but you do not need to study all three degrees in order to do self-healing. The First Degree is enough to teach you simple, but very effective self-help techniques. First Degree Reiki can be learned in a weekend workshop. Consider having your significant other also learn Reiki so that you can exchange Reiki treatments.

POLARITY THERAPY

Theory and Technique

Polarity therapy is another form of hands-on healing energy work. In a typical session the practitioner places his hands on different defined points on the body, depending on the pain issue, and holds them in place for a certain period of time. Massage and pressing on various body points may also be used.

References

A Guide to Polarity Therapy: The Gentle Art of Hands on Healing by Martin Seidman
Your Healing Hands: The Polarity Experience by Richard Gordon

Referrals

Polarity Wellness Center
10 Leonard Street, Suite A
New York, N.Y. 10013
(212) 334- 8392.

Self Help

There is an excellent polarity self-help manual, *Polarity for the People, The Handbook,* by Patricia M. Curit, with a number of exercises and self help techniques. This publication can be ordered from her at:

Patricia M. Curit
P. O. Box 2283
Durango, CO 81301

VIBRATIONAL HEALING MASSAGE THERAPY

Theory and Technique

Vibrational healing massage therapy is a leading edge body-work that works with the physical structure and emotions to free up tensions and stresses held in the body. This can include reawakening the nervous system, restoring circulation to injured areas, and letting go of chronic pain or stiffness. There are approximately 16 basic techniques that align, loosen, and connect the body so that tensions can reverberate freely. Special sensitive stretching, rebounding, and torquing are some of the techniques allowing the energy to flow again. This therapy is energizing because the techniques release the most "congested" areas of the body first.

References

A *Vibrational Healing Massage Manual,* a video tape, and a set of audio tapes are available from

> World School of Massage
> 401 32nd Ave
> San Francisco, CA 94121
> (415) 221-2533.

Referrals

Referrals can be obtained from the World School of Massage. If you live in the San Francisco Bay Area, the founder of this therapy and Director of the World School, Patricia Cramer, is available for consultation.

CHI-GUNG

Theory and Technique

Chi-gung is a self-help form of energy work that emphasizes movement, self-massage, breathing, and forms of meditation to balance and circulate *chi.* Basically it is an exercise system that is practiced throughout China. It has gained wide popularity in the West and classes are generally available in large American cities. Many research studies have documented its effectiveness in curing and alleviating symptoms of illness. There are many forms of Chi-gung practiced today. Instruction from a qualified teacher or self-instruction from a video is required. Do not necessarily expect immediate results, rather it is the long term practice which results in pain relief and healing.

References

Books:
  The Complete System of Self Healing: Internal Exercises by Stephen T. Chang
  Chi Self Massage by Mantak Chia

Vital Energy, Easy Oriental Exercises for Health and Well Being, by Jacqueline Young
Video:
QiGong for Health—an excellent two-tape series that explains the warm-up and exercise routine in a clear manner.

Referrals

American Foundation of Traditional Chinese Medicine
505 Beach St., San Francisco, CA 94133
(415) 776-0502

CHAPTER 23

ICE, HEAT, HERBAL COMPRESSES, SALT AND ESSENTIAL OIL BATHS, SALVES AND OINTMENTS

Introduction

COLD AND HEAT, herbal compresses, as well as various herbal, essential oil, and salt baths have played an important role in relieving pain since antiquity. Everyone will react differently to each of these modalities. Therefore, we present a summary of each method for you to try each out and see what works. Indeed, various combinations may work best.

COLD THERAPY

What Is It?

Cold therapy is the application of ice or a commercial cold gel pack to painful points on the body. Usually the skin is protected by putting the ice or gel pack in a towel or cloth before application.

Why Does It Work?

Cold therapy numbs the nerve endings and decreases the blood supply to the area where cold is applied. It is particularly helpful during the first 48 hours after an injury because it reduces inflammation and swelling. Some have found it helpful after the initial 48 hours and prefer it over heat. However, cold therapy can be irritating because its application may tense the area up and tighten the muscles, resulting in more contractions and pain. Be sure to test your reaction. If cold therapy does not help, avoid it.

How Is It Applied?

Cold therapy can be applied with a commercial flexible gel pack, with ice cubes in a plastic bag, a bag of frozen peas or frozen rice, or an ice massage.

For ice massage, freeze water in a paper cup, and apply it by massaging the painful area. Massage should last about 3 to 5 minutes. The gel packs or ice cubes in towels should be used around 15-20 minutes. Enhance the effectiveness of cold therapy with visualization by imagining that the ice is freezing pain signals so that they cannot be transmitted to the brain.

HEAT THERAPY

What Is It?

Heat therapy is the application of moist heat, dry heat, infra-red heat, or heated herbs to the painful area.

Why Does It Work?

Heat, especially moist and infrared heat, is effective in pain relief because it relaxes muscle spasms, relieves stiffness, brings blood and oxygen to the painful areas, and promotes overall relaxation. Heated herbal packs also bring the power of healing herbs to the injured area.

How Is Heat Applied?

There are many ways to apply heat to the back. Examine the methods listed below:

• Electric Heating Pads Without Moist Heat: Great for in the office or away from home, where moist heat would be impractical. Try 10 to 15 minutes at low to medium heat. Do not use if inflammation is present or the injury is recent.

• Electric Heating Pads With Moist Heat: Moist heat is the preferable way to go because it penetrates more deeply. Most commercial heating pads have a moist heat option, a thin sheet of a sponge-like material you dampen. Place the heating pad against the back at low to medium temperature for about 15 to 20 minutes. It loosens tight muscles. Try 20 minutes in the morning, 20 minutes at lunch and 20 minutes after dinner.

• Hydrocolaters: These packs, available at any drug store, contain a gel material in a canvas pack. Heat them in boiling water and apply them to the back with a few layers of towels in between. They are good because this moist heat retains its temperature for nearly a half an hour. Apply it to the back for 10 to 15 minutes.

• Microwave Gel Packs: Available at any drug store, these can be heated in a microwave oven and applied over the sore area with a towel buffer for the time designated on the pack

• Moist Warm Towels: Moist heat can also be applied by soaking towels in hot water, wringing them out and applying to the back for three minutes at a time. You may need someone to assist with application. A variant of this would be to alternate warm moist towels and cold moist towels, applying each for three minutes.

• Warm Baths or Pulsating Showers: Lying in a warm bath or sitting on a stool, or standing in the shower with warm water gently pounding on the back is another excellent way to loosen tight muscles. Try these methods for 15 to 20 minutes at a time.

• Hot Tubs and Whirlpool Baths: For those lucky enough to own a hot tub, take advantage of the warm water and pulsating jets for about ten to fifteen minutes. Make sure the water temperature is not above 100 degrees because higher temperatures can actually cause muscle spasms. Usually for less than $100.00 you can purchase a device that will give the bath tub the massage/pulsating effects that a true hot tub can give. Such a device is well worth the investment.

• Infrared Heat: Infrared heat is highly effective in relieving sore muscles and muscle spasms. An excellent hand-held infrared heat therapy instrument (the infralume health therapy instrument) can be purchased for $24.95 from Nordic Track mail order. Call 1-800-445-2606. Another excellent infrared product is the Thermotex heating pad which uses infrared heat to deeply penetrate the muscles. It can be ordered from Thermotex in Calgary, Canada.

Enhance the Healing Power of Water With Visualization

Warm water is highly relaxing and also relieves pain caused by tense muscles. You can increase the pain-relieving power of the water by using the visualization techniques discussed in Chapter 6.

Enhance the Healing Power of Water With a
Back-U-Pressure Device and Exercise

In *Hot Water Therapy* by Horay and Harp, excellent exercise routines as well as massage techniques are discussed. We believe it is a must-have book in any back pain sufferer's library. The authors describe how to make an excellent massage tool they call a back-u-pressure device. It requires two tennis balls, two sturdy rubber bands and a towel 30 inches long or an old pair of panty-hose. Put the balls in the center of the towel or pantyhose (after cutting one leg off, slide the balls into the knee area), roll the towel length wise to tighten so a long tube is formed (no need to roll the pantyhose), and place the rubber bands by the outer ends of each ball on the towel or pantyhose to keep the balls in place. You now have made a back-u-pressure device. Use the device by holding each end of the towel or pantyhose with your arms such that the balls are against the back. Lean into the balls against a shower wall and feel for tender points. Once one is found lightly press into it for 30 to 60 seconds until tenderness disappears and remove the device. You probably have hit a pressure point. The pain should go away from that area. Also use it as a massage device for the lower and upper back. Make sure each ball lies on a different side of the spinal column.

Most traditional back exercises can be done in a bath tub or hot tub. *Hot Water Therapy* contains excellent exercise and stretching routines which can easily be done in hot water. Try them out.

HERBAL PACK THERAPY

What Is It?
Herbal packs look like small cushions and contain a variety of healing herbs including yucca and cinnamon. They can be worn on the back.

Why Do They Work?
Generally a typical herbal pack up can be heated in a microwave oven for about three minutes and then applied to the sore area of the back. The special combination of herbs makes you sweat in the area of application, and the healing herbs penetrate the sore areas.

How Does One Apply An Herbal Pack?
Most herbal packs come with detailed instructions. After heating in a microwave oven for about three minutes on high, apply the herbal pack for about 15 to 20 minutes to the stiff or painful area. The pack loosens tight muscles, brings oxygenated blood into the area, and the herb application speeds pain-relief and assists the healing process.

EPSOM SALT AND HERBAL AND ESSENTIAL OIL BATHS

What Are They?

For these types of baths, Epsom salt, herbs, or essential oils are added to regular warm water bath.

Why Do They Work?

Epsom salt baths are highly effective because they induce sweating, allowing the body to release various toxins. The effect of herbal and essential oil baths depends on the type of herb or oil added to the bath. Certain herbs and oils promote circulation, while others relax muscles and nerves.

How are Epsom Salt, Herbal and Essential Oil Baths Prepared and How Long Should They Be Used?

Epsom salts baths are prepared by adding two large handfuls of Epsom salts to normal warm bath water and soaking for as long as 20 minutes. Be prepared to sweat. Have a cold compress nearby to place on the forehead in case of dizziness. When ready to leave the bath, rinse the body down with a cool sponge or washcloth to close the pores.

Herbal baths are prepared by adding herbs to warm bath water through liquid extracts, powdered dry herbs, or by placing the herbs in a cheesecloth bag, running the bath water through the cloth and then placing the cheesecloth directly in the water. Concentrated oils of medicinal herbs can also be added to warm bath water. Due to their heavy concentration, only a few drops of these oils need to be added. Follow the directions on the commercially prepared herbs for use in a warm water bath. Herbs that relax muscles and calm nerves include chamomile, lime flowers, and catnip.

Essential oils are very concentrated oils extracted from plants and flowers. Only a few drops of essential oils in a bath are necessary due to their heavy concentration Effective essential oils include lavender, bay, rosemary, pine and basil. Soak in herbal or essential oil baths for 20 minutes.

Oat or wheat bran baths cleanse and relax. Two handfuls of either oat or wheat bran mixed in water will help a great deal.

HERBAL COMPRESSES, PLASTERS, AND PASTES

What Are They?

Herbal compresses are made up of gauze or cheesecloth bags containing herbs, and applied to the skin. Herbal plasters are ointments prepared with the herb in a wax base so that the herb adheres to the skin. Similarly, herbs can be applied by mixing the dry herb or crushed leaves with hot water and flour, cornmeal, or bran to form a paste. Herbs can be purchased at a local health products store.

Why Do they Work?

Herbal compresses, pastes and plasters work because of the herb's healing power and because they are applied directly to the affected area. Herbs that are ideal for plasters that relieve strain and stiffness include cayenne pepper (capsicum), ginger and lobelia.

How Are Compresses, Pastes, and Plasters Applied?

After preparing the compress, paste, or plaster, it should be applied directly to the sore area. Compresses should normally be left on for about 20 minutes. Pastes or plasters can be left on for hours. Back plasters are normally available in drug stores.

SALVES AND OINTMENTS

What Are They?

We've all seen the commercial salves and ointments for pain relief, such as Ben Gay. There are also commercial homeopathic ointments for pain relief.

Why Do They Work?

Ointments and salves work because of their properties and because they remain in constant contact with the body. Perhaps the most popular pain relieving ointments are those that contain menthol and eucalyptus oil. These ointments, classified as counter-irritants, provide a heat or warm sensation which in essence distracts you from the pain by substituting a different sensation. *For those with fibromyalgia, we recommend staying away from them.* Other commercial ointments contain typically 10% salycin mixed in with a mineral oil base. Homeopathic formulas typically contain arnica cream or ruta cream mixed in with beeswax or lanolin oil.

Capsacin cream or Ointment: There are a number of creams or ointments that contain .25 or .75 per cent capsacin. These are effective in reducing pain if used continuously. Initially they may cause a burning sensation, but with continued use, the burning sensation abates. These ointments can be highly effective.

Penetran: This is a new over-the-counter product containing a strong ammonia solution, also highly effective in relieving pain.

How Are They Used?

Apply the ointment or salve to the painful area and follow the directions on the box.

CHAPTER 24

AROMATHERAPY: USING ESSENTIAL OILS FOR PAIN RELIEF, RELAXATION, AND CHANGING MOOD

What Is Aromatherapy?

Aromatherapy involves the use of essential oils obtained from herbs, plants, and flowers to treat numerous diseases and painful conditions. These oils are extremely powerful and are used widely in France, Germany, and England. Various essential oils have the following strong medicinal properties: antiviral, antibacterial, antispasmodic, anti-inflammatory, sedating, energizing, pain relieving, and mood enhancing. They are especially powerful in relieving back pain due to their antispasmodic, mood altering, and pain relieving effects.

Why Does Aromatherapy Work?

Our body can receive essential oils in two ways: 1. inhaling the aroma of the oil, affecting the olfactory nerves and portions of the brain, or 2. by direct application of the oil to the skin, so that the oil is absorbed into the blood stream through the capillaries, eventually affecting the brain. Depending on the oil or the mixture of oils, various physiological or psychological effects are produced. For instance, psychologically, the direct application of jasmine mixed with a carrier oil is calming and euphoric. In contrast, the direct application of half a drop of peppermint oil to each temple energizes and stimulates. Physiologically, such oils as eucalyptus and clary sage mixed with a carrier oil relieve muscle spasms when applied to the affected muscle.

When Do You Use Aromatherapy?

Use aromatherapy daily. Try these suggestions based on desired effect. To relieve soreness and stiffness, apply aromatherapy blends prior to bed time, after a morning shower, before and after exercising, and any other time during the time that you develop pain or stiffness. For mood enhancement, apply the mood-lifting blends in the morning and other times during the day when you need a pick-me-up.

How Do You Prepare and Use Essential Oils?

As an overview, we will discuss: 1. essential supplies and measurements; 2. essential oils for relieving back pain and anxiety associated with it; 3. carrier oils; 4. methods of application of essential oils; 5. how to make formulas; and 6. suggested formulas. With this information you can make formulas and find which combinations of essential oils are most effective in treating back pain.

Essential Supplies

- One 4 or 8 oz. dark bottle to mix the oil blends.
- A dropper to measure drops of essential oils.
- A measuring cup that measures liquid ounces.
- Four dark 2 ounce bottles and tops to store the blends.
- 8 ounces of favorite carrier oil.
- High quality pure essential oils to use in the blends.
- Paper towels or rags to use in cleaning.
- Stick-on labels to label the blends.

Essential Measurements

Certain essential oils may be applied directly to the skin. In this case the measurement is a drop; for instance apply one drop of peppermint oil to the temples. Essential oils come in small dark jars with a top to measure drops. A drop is equal to 25 milligrams.

- One ml. or milliliter is equivalent to 25-30 drops.
- 30 ml. is equal to one ounce.
- 15 ml. is equal to a tablespoon.

Essential oils are strong and generally need to be diluted in a carrier oil. Carrier oils are measured in terms of milliliters. There will always be more of a carrier oil in a formula than an essential oil.

As a general rule there should be no more than 15 drops of one oil or a combination of oils in 15 ml. of a carrier oil. While the number of drops can be raised to assure a higher potency or effect, it should never be more than 30 drops. We recommend that it be no higher than 20 drops per 15 ml.

Essential Oils

It is extremely important to purchase high quality essential oils. Most of the oils discussed in this chapter can be purchased for $9-$15.00 for about $3/4$ of an ounce. However, these oils last a long time because such a tiny amount of oil is used in a blend. Quality is very important, so we recommend discussing the quality of the oil with the vendor. Make sure that the oil is pure, not diluted. However, jasmine absolute is very expensive, so we recommend that it be purchased in a dilution since jasmine is still highly effective even when diluted. Essential oils will be listed by their physiological or psychological effect. A plus sign marks a highly effective oil.

Pain Relief	Antispasmodic	Calming	Mood Elevating
Clove+	Marjoram	Blue Chamomile	Jasmine+
Birch+	Clary Sage	Neroli	Clary Sage
Blue Chamomile+	Geranium	Lavendar	Rosemary
Peppermint	Ginger	Eucalyptus	Ylang Ylang
Lavendar			
Oregano			

Carrier Oils

Carrier oils are the base oil the essential oils are mixed with to make an appropriate blend. We recommend the following carrier oils, based on their properties and cost.

• Sweet Almond Oil: This medium weight oil is relatively inexpensive. As it is lubricating rather than penetrating, it is an excellent choice for massage blends.

• Jojoba Oil: This oil is highly stable and is highly resistant to rancidity. While higher priced than sweet almond oil, it is very effective for dry, mature, or oily skin.

• Sesame Oil: This oil is moderate in price, highly resistant to rancidity and deeply penetrating, making it ideal for pain relief. Sesame oil can be purchased in the vegetable oil section of the supermarket or in a health food store. Make sure the oil is cold pressed. Do not buy toasted sesame oil, which is used as a seasoning in Asian cooking.

Methods of Application

The following table suggests the number of drops to be used for various applications and the amount of carrier oil to be included.

Application	Number of Drops of Essential Oil	Amount of Carrier Oil
Massage oil	50-60	120 ml.
Lotion	50-60	120 ml.
Ointment	50-60	60 ml.
Topical	50-60	30 ml.
Compress	10	4 oz. water
Bath	10-15	tub of water

These measurements can be adjusted downward. For instance, if you only want to make one ounce or 30 ml. of a massage oil, that would be 25 per cent of 120 ml. or 30 ml. In terms of drops, that would also be 25 per cent of the suggested dosage or 15 drops.

• Direct: Place a drop or two directly on the skin. Make sure the oil is not a skin irritant.

• Direct in a Blend: Prepare a formula and then lightly rub into the skin.

• Massage: Deeply rub a blend into the skin.

• Compress

• Bath

• Diffuse in Air-purchase an electrical diffuser.

• Lotion

How To A Make Your Own Blends

Making your own formulas or blends is very easy. Gather the supplies, including dropper, a mixing bottle, a storage bottle, and the carrier and essential oils required. First pour a little less of the carrier oil than is needed into the mixing bottle so there is room for the essential oils to be added. Second, place the number of drops of the first essential oil into the mixing bottle with the carrier oil. Then mix the essential oil with the carrier oil by placing the top on the mixing bottle and shaking the bottle. Third, clean the dropper. Fourth, extract the number of drops required for the second essential oil and place it in the mixing bottle and then mix the second essential oil with the carrier and first essential oil. Follow this procedure until all the required essential oils are mixed with the carrier oil. Finally, write on the label the type of blend (i.e. muscle soreness), the blend formula, and then place the label on the bottle and place scotch tape over the label to protect it from drips of blended oils.

You can make our recommended blends or purchase books with recommendations for blends.

Recommended Direct Applications and Formulas

Listed below are some recommended direct applications or formulas. They are listed by psychological or physiological effect they produce. All blends assume that a total one ounce blend will be produced. To make a two-ounce blend, double the number of drops and carrier oil; to make a four-ounce blend, multiply by four the formula requirements. Each of us is unique; one formula may work well on one person, but not on another, so experimentation is expected. Mix the essential oils together with the carrier oil according to the desired psychological or physiological effect and determine the right blend.

Calming

• Directly apply one drop of pure lavender oil to each temple, under the nose and on each wrist.

• Formula: Massage into neck, shoulders, and arms.

> 1 oz. carrier oil
> 10 drops neroli
> 10 drops lavender
> 10 drops ylang-ylang

Relief of Muscle Pain, Stiffness and Soreness

• Formula: Massage into area of stiffness and pain.

> 1 oz. carrier oil
> 10 drops of rosemary
> 10 drops of lavender
> 10 drops of marjoram

• Formula: Massage into area of stiffness and pain.

> 1 oz. carrier oil
> 10 drops of eucalyptus
> 10 drops of pine
> 10 drops of anise seed

Mood Elevating

• Direct Application: Apply one drop each of ylang-ylang or jasmine to temples, behind each ear, on each wrist, and under the nose.

• Formula: Massage into back of neck, shoulder area and arms.

> 1 oz carrier oil
> 10 drops ylang-ylang
> 10 drops patchouli
> 5 drops jasmine

Other Formulas

There are a number of excellent aromatherapy books with quite a large number of formulas organized by desired effect. They include:

> *Aromatherapy Workbook* by Marcel Lavabre
> *500 Formulas for Aromatherapy by* Carol & David Schiller

CHAPTER 25

SELF-MASSAGE, VIBRATION, AND ELECTRICAL STIMULATION

IN THIS CHAPTER, we present different ways to stimulate the body physically for pain relief. The methods include hands-on techniques such as massage and methods requiring a device such as a vibrator or other electrical source of stimulation. All these techniques work on the gate theory of pain relief--that is, shutting down the gate to pain by interrupting the pain signal's transmission to the brain.

SELF-MASSAGE

What Is It?
Massage is the stroking, gentle rubbing, kneading, light pounding, or other touch techniques on muscles, tendons, or other soft tissue. A professional massage therapist is an option, but self-massage is easy, provides great relief, and can be done in the privacy of your own home.

Why Does It Work?
Massage is excellent for pain relief because it distracts one from pain, calms the nerves, and focuses the mind on pleasurable sensations. Massage benefits the body and mind in several ways. It improves circulation of blood and lymph, relaxes and loosens tight muscles, aids the elimination of waste products from the muscles, stimulates acupressure points, and also relieves anxiety and stress.

Before commencing any massage program, *check with your physician* to ensure that it will not be harmful. Generally, if the pain is a muscular problem, not a structural problem, massage will be fine.

How Do You Do It?

You will need the following items:

• A light exercise mat, covered in vinyl or a towel to absorb massage oil.

• A pillow.

• A massage oil, preferably a vegetable oil mixed with an essential oil such as chamomile or lavender. While these mixed oils can be purchased commercially, you can make massage oils by combining a carrier oil, such as sweet almond oil or a penetrating oil like sesame, with the above or other essential oils. See Chapter 24 on Aromatherapy for detailed instructions.

• An incense holder and incense to enrich the experience.

• Soothing music.

• Low lights and a few lit candles.

• A warm, private place. Obviously, you may have to remove some or all clothing for self-massage, so make sure the room is warm, comfortable, and appropriately private. A chill will cause muscles to tense up.

Oil Application

Massage oil should be used because it will eliminate the resistance of skin on skin and facilitate smooth strokes. Place the oil in both palms, rub them together to disperse and warm the oil, and then lightly stroke the oil on the parts of the body to be massaged. Repeat this process when more oil is needed.

The Massage Strokes

The following strokes can be used in self-massage with either one or both hands. Experiment with the following techniques to find the most pleasant and effective for your needs.

Effleurage: Stroking with the palms open in any direction in a rhythmic manner.

Pettrisage: Deep movements that involve picking up the flesh and muscles as well squeezing and rolling them.

Pressure: Using fingers, or thumbs or heels of the hands to make straight penetrating or circular penetrating movements on the flesh and muscles.

Percussion: Lightly pounding the body with the fists, tapping the body with open hands, or hitting the body with the sides of the hands.

The Massage

Using the selected strokes, massage the areas that are tight and tense, or if possible, do a full body massage for total relaxation. It is generally best to start at one end of the body and gently proceed to the rest of the body. For instance, start at the head, proceed to the shoulders and neck, then to the arms, chest, upper back, abdomen, lower back, hips, thighs, and remainder of the legs and feet. *Pay close attention to tight muscles in the thighs as these muscles are often responsible for much back pain.* Once you have a routine set, you may want to tape record it.

Don't forget the importance of deep breathing during self-massage. Deep breathing helps release toxins and promotes full relaxation.

Self-massage techniques are covered in a number of books. You may also consult *The Complete Book of Massage* by Clare Maxwell Hudson for excellent full body, facial, and neck self-massage routines. If you are interested in being more proficient, attend massage classes or watch massage videos available in the library or video rental store.

Self-Massage Routine

We are grateful to Marie Carbone of the National Holistic Institute of Emeryville, California for the following self-massage routine.

Using the guidelines above for setting, clothing, room temperature, etc., follow these steps for a relaxing, healthful self-massge.

1. Pre-Massage:

All movements should be smooth, slow, and gentle. Stretch your arms up overhead 2-3 times. Shrug your shoulders up and down 2-3 times and then circle the shoulders backward and forward 2-3 times. Squeeze the shoulder blades together with elbows bent, and then once again with arms extended behind. Nod head forward gently, bringing chin towards chest 2-3 times. Arch head and neck back gently 2-3 times. Bend head to each side gently, moving the ear towards the shoulder. Do 2-3 sitting cat stretches—arching the belly out and then rounding out the spine. Grab right elbow with left hand and twist at the waist and then grab the left elbow with the right hand and twist again. Extend the legs out and point and flex the feet 2-3 times. Circle the ankles clockwise and then counter-clockwise. Finally, stand up and shake everything out gently. Now you're ready for the massage.

2. The Face Massage:

Palms facing in, gently stroke both hands across the forehead 2-3 times. Stroke across the eye area 2-3 times. With thumb, press the bone in the eye arch on the inside end of the eyebrows for several seconds. Massage temples, paying attention to sore points. Squeeze outside of ears and then inside. Gently flick the ears with the fingertips. Finish with a scalp rub, vigorously rubbing the scalp all over with the fingertips.

3. The Neck:

With both hands, squeeze up and down the back of the neck 2-3 times. With the thumbs, massage in circular motion the indentations at the base of the skull where it meets the neck.

4. The Hands and Arms:

Squeeze and gently twist the flesh of the arms from shoulder to wrist 2-3 times. Squeeze and knead the hands gently. Press web between thumb and forefinger with thumb and forefinger of opposite hand, or use your elbow to massage the point.

5. The Back:

Make fists and with the thumb knuckle, massage in circles over the kidney area. The move down to the back of the waist, closer to the hip bones and massage any sore points.

6. The Legs and Feet:

Knead the upper thighs and then calves. Bend each toe down and pull gently on each toe. Use opposite heel to massage over and around the instep on top of each foot. Squeeze each foot in your hands. Grab the toes on each foot and squeeze them together. Finally, tap and slap all over both feet.

Professional Massages: A Few Important Tips

While self-massage is wonderful, at some point you may wish to seek the services of a bodyworker for a full professional massage. If so, here are some tips for choosing the right one.

• Choose a massage therapist by referral and reputation, not the phone book. Ask friends, relatives, your physician or physical therapist for names of reputable bodyworkers in the area.

• Think about gender. Would a same sex therapist be more comfortable, or would gender not be an issue? This is something to consider before choosing a bodyworker.

• Be sure that the bodyworker/therapist is certified and has had sufficient education and experience in massage.

• Explain your condition and discuss the type of massage the bodyworker believes is appropriate.

• Do not let the bodyworker do anything that hurts or doesn't feel right. Speak up if he or she is pressing to hard or doing anything else that doesn't feel good.

• Discuss the fee and time limits of the massage *beforehand.*

• Discuss the setting and type of oil to be used.

• Never massage areas where there is infection or inflammation.

VIBRATION

What is It?
Vibration can be induced on the body by rapid movement of hands, by a skilled bodyworker, or a commercial vibrating machine.

Why Does It Work?
Vibration relieves pain for a number of reasons. First it distracts; second, through sufficiently strong and continued action, pain circuits are overridden; third, circulation is improved, resulting in the elimination of waste products and lactic acid from the muscles.

Equipment
Commercial hand-held massagers and vibrators range in price from $20.00 to over $100.00. At a minimum, the equipment should have at least two speeds (high and low), a large ribbed surface, and a small pinpoint area for massaging specific spots or acupressure points.

Good sources for excellent massagers include Brookstone retail stores, the Sharper Image mail order catalog, and holistic health fairs. Try massagers out and decide which is most effective and comfortable.

How To Use Mechanical Massage Equipment
Hand-held massagers should be applied *carefully* and discussed with your physician before use. As a matter of general caution, we suggest that a mechanical massager not be applied directly over the painful area at first, but more to the side of the area. Doing this will accustom the body to it, and eventually, application to the site of the pain should be possible. The literature suggests that for vibration to be effective, it should be applied for 30-45 minutes.

However, each one of us is different, so experiment. Follow the directions that come with the equipment.

Massagers can also be applied to various trigger points on the body to relieve back pain. Trigger points are shown in the following illustration. You may also want to massage the healing points noted in Chapter 21.

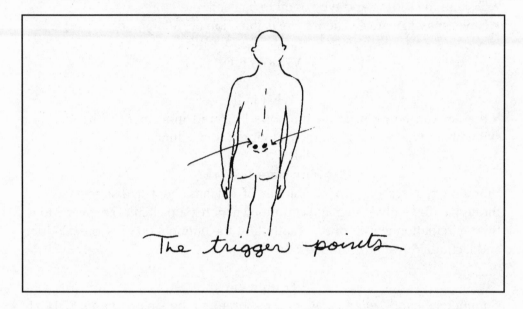

The trigger points

ELECTRICAL STIMULATION WITH A TENS UNIT

What Is It?

TENS stands for "trans subcutaneous electrical nerve stimulation." A TENS unit is a medical device containing a 9-volt battery, with adjustable controls to vary the frequency and pulsation of electrical current, and connected to wires linked to electrodes that can be placed on various spots on the body to relieve pain.

Why Does it Work?

A TENS unit works on the theory that the application of electrical signals to certain spots on the body can block the pain message and allow endorphins to be released. In some sense a TENS unit works like vibration, heat, or ice. TENS units have had mixed results in chronic back pain patients. Sometimes they are very effective with certain individuals, but not with others. A TENS unit may work for you, so discuss the possible use of TENS therapy with your physician and give it a try. It is a prescription medical device normally covered by insurance.

How Do You Use It?

The difficulty with a TENS unit is learning where to place the electrodes and how to adjust the intensity, rate, and quality of the pulsating electricity. Do not rely on the instructions alone. Have a qualified physical therapist instruct you in its use, including the proper placement of the electrodes. Follow these tips also.

• Adjust the current so that it is comfortable. Do not put the unit on full power. Experiment with the different electrical settings to see which adjustments of the electrical current give the most pain relief.

• Some physicians or therapists suggest that the electrodes should be placed over the painful area; others suggest along the spinal cord, while others suggest that the electrodes should be placed so that a line can be drawn through the painful area from one electrode to another. You might even experiment in placing the TENS unit over various acupressure points.

• Combine TENS therapy with other forms of pain relief such as deep breathing, healing point therapy, music or humor therapy. Indeed, try visualizing that the electrical impulses are releasing endorphins while the current is pulsating. (From *The Back Pain Book: A Self-Help Guide for the Daily Relief of Back and Neck Pain*, by Mike Hage, from Peachtree Publishers.)

• Do *not* keep the unit on continuously. Use it for a maximum of $1^1/_2$ hours and assess the results. If the pain is gone, leave it off until the pain returns. This is especially important because the electrical impulse can become very annoying, thus less effective, and you may lose confidence in the device. (From *The Back Pain Book: A Self-Help Guide for the Daily Relief of Back and Neck Pain* by Mike Hage.)

Other Electrical Devices

There are a number of other portable devices on the market that stimulate acupressure points with a short or continuous charge of electricity.

The following products can be ordered from the Lifestyle Fascination Catalog by phoning 800- 669-0987

• Crystaldyne Pain Zapper (short charge)

• Electro-Acupuncture (continuous charge)

• Acustim Personal Wellness Stimulator (short charge)

CHAPTER 26

UNCONTRACTING MUSCLES: THE FOLD AND HOLD & TOUCH FOR HEALTH TECHNIQUES

DURING ROBERT MILLER'S TREATMENT, research, and schooling, he learned many effective techniques to *immediately* reduce or eliminate pain in the back region and in associated muscles. The following techniques take time and patience to learn; however, *they are extremely powerful*—their mastery can result in prompt pain reduction and/or relief.

Uncontracting Muscles

Most back pain is caused by contracted or shortened muscles in the lower, middle, or upper back, as well as those in the thighs and legs. Once you discover those in contraction, and successfully uncontract them, pain will be significantly lessened or eliminated.

Identifying Contracted Muscles

Follow these steps to locate and document shortened muscles:

1. Feel the area of pain: Place a hand lightly over the area of pain. If the tissue feels hard or board like, then the muscles in that area are contracted and probably in spasm. Note the location and write it down to help you remember where it is.

2. Touch the muscles on the legs: Lightly touch and rub the muscles on the front, back, and sides of the legs and thighs. Note any muscles that feel hard.

3. Examine lower back and buttocks: Lightly touch the buttocks and low back areas, including those near the spine, and note any areas of tightness.

4. Touch middle, upper back, shoulder, and neck areas—write down any areas of tightness or restriction.

5. Lie on the back: If it softens and comes into full contact with the floor, all the muscles are loose. Lightly touch the hard areas of the back that do not make full contact with the floor and note them.

Once the contracted muscles are located, use one or more of the following methods to uncontract tight muscles:

Techniques to Uncontract Muscles: Introduction

These techniques are discussed in detail in the Fold and Hold and Touch for Health sections. Fold and Hold can provide dramatic relief, and works primarily on large muscle groups by deeply relaxing the muscle in spasm, followed by gentle stretching. Touch for Health techniques reduce muscle spasms by clearing blocked energy in the body. Particular attention should be paid to the massage techniques to release spasms and weaken overly tight muscles. *Obtain your doctor's approval before using these techniques.*

Increasing the Contraction to Uncontract the Muscle

While this technique cannot be used with every contracted muscle, it is effective because further contraction of the muscle puts it to sleep and then it is gently stretched out. For example, if there is tightness, stiffness, and pain in the center of the back slightly up from the hip bone, follow these steps:

1. Further contract the muscle: Place the hands on the buttocks and gently lean backward to move further into the contraction. Remain in the further contracted position for one to two minutes.

2. Stretch forward: Gently and slowly stretch out of the further contraction by leaning forward.

Finding Positions That Relieve Pain

This technique involves some slight experimentation with the legs, hips, pelvis area, and upper torso. *Be very gentle with yourself* and do not stretch or move anything in a sudden or jerky manner. *Do not move into pain.* The concept is to adjust the body to an ideal position that relieves pain and/or uncontracts muscles. Follow these steps:

1. Adjusting the legs and feet:

Contracted or tight muscles in the legs have a major effect on the back muscles. Stand up straight with the knees slightly bent. First rotate the left foot and then the right inward and then outward. If either movement helps relieve pain, note down the effective movement. Then move each leg out to the front, then to the sides, and then to the back. If any movement helps relieve pain, note it down. Place one foot behind the other and vice versa and if any movement relieves pain note it. While still standing, grab the left ankle and lightly pull back, let it down, and then do the same with the right ankle. If *any* action relieves pain, note it. Move the legs and feet in other directions and if pain is relieved, again, note it. Once you have moved the legs and thighs in all possible directions and found where relief was obtained, you have located an ideal position of comfort for the legs.

2. *Adjusting the hip and pelvis areas:*

Next, test the hip and pelvis area in both standing and sitting positions. First stand and move the pelvis forward by tucking in the tummy, tightening the abdominal muscles, and moving the buttocks forward by rotating the hips forward, making sure the spine is erect and shoulders back. Then move the pelvis backward and slightly to each side. Repeat the same process while sitting on the in a chair. Note in what positions pain relief is obtained. Generally, rotation of the pelvis forward helps reduce back pain.

3. *Adjusting the mid and upper back:*

In standing and sitting positions test the upper torso by leaning forward, then backward and to each side with the shoulders back and spine straight. Note the position that affords the most comfort.

4. *Adjusting arms:*

Hold both arms out to the sides, move them up and down, back and forth, noting positions that decrease discomfort.

5. *Adjusting neck and shoulders:*

Turn the neck gently side to side, bend it forward and back, and shrug the shoulders up and down, again noting positions that provide relief.

By rechecking your notes, you will find the most comfortable positions for the legs, pelvis and upper torso. Place yourself in that position for standing and sitting and see what combination offers the most relief. Remember be gentle and do not go to extremes. Do not assume any position that is painful.

Stretching Away from Tightness

Another effective method to immediately relieve pain is to stretch gently away from the tightness. For example, if there is pain in the center of the lower back, gently stretch forward so that the muscle is stretched. Do not stretch to any extreme. Hold it for a short period of time.

Placing Energized Hands Over the Area of Pain

Rub both hands together in a brisk fashion until they are warm. Then place the warm hand or hands directly over the area of pain. It is not necessary to touch the body. This method balances out energy in the sore muscle.

The *Fold and Hold* Method for Uncontracting Muscles and Relieving Pain
One of the most effective methods to immediately relieve muscle pain caused by spasm is "Fold and Hold" as described by Dr. Dale Anderson. This mobilization method is a "user friendly" modification of the Strain/Counter Strain manipulation technique developed by Lawrence Jones. The material in this section is adapted from Dr. Anderson's excellent book *Muscle Pain Relief in 90 Seconds—The Fold and Hold Method.* It is a "must have" in any chronic back pain sufferer's library.

Dr. Anderson defines mobilization as "helping the body find positions where it can move and function efficiently." Its goal, he maintains, is "to remold and reposition the body in a way that restores normal body function and movement, thereby relieving pain."

Fold and Hold operates on the theory that pain is caused by muscle spasm. A muscle in spasm is shortened and contains tender spots. Additional discomfort from a spastic muscle can occur in three ways: 1. touching tender spots; 2. working or loading the muscle in an active manner; and 3. stretching, pulling or lengthening the muscle in a passive manner. The theory behind Fold and Hold is to first deeply relax the spastic muscle by putting it to sleep, gradually reawaken it, and then stretch and eventually strengthen it. The general steps described below are then followed by specific instructions.

1. Find the Tender Spot: Muscles in spasm are generally located at the area of discomfort, and can be tight and hard. Within that area, feel for the real tender or "ouch" spot. Find it by using the index and middle fingers pressing over the painful area, until a very tender spot is felt. In most cases the tender spot will be in the area of discomfort, though in a small number of instances the tender spot will be on the opposite side of the body from the pain. There may be multiple tender spots. In this case work on one tender spot at a time.

2. Fold the Body Over the Tender Spot or Find a Comfortable Position: Muscles are taken out of spasm by shortening and then relaxing them. "Fold" the appropriate part of the body over the tender spot until the pain is eliminated. Pain goes away when the spastic muscle is put to sleep by placing it in "a shortened, relaxed and comfortable position." In doing this you need to "fine tune" the position. Monitor the tender spot with the fingers, and adjust the body position so that the pain in the tender spot goes away.

3. Hold Comfortable Position 90 Seconds: Once you are in the comfortable or treatment position, accomplish pain relief by maintaining that position for a minimum of 90 seconds. If you have fingers on the tender spot you will note that it melts as the pain goes away. You may want to remain in the position for about 2 to $2^1/_2$ minutes.

4. Return to Normal Position: Once the muscle is put to sleep, do not return to the normal position too fast. Awaken the muscle *slowly*, and *gently* return to the unfolded or normal position.

5. Stretch and Strengthen: While not part of the Fold and Hold routine, to avoid future problems, you need to stretch the spastic muscle that was treated, as well as stretch the tight connective tissue surrounding that muscle, and then strengthen these muscles.

The above explains the general theory surrounding this excellent technique. Now let's get specific and discuss how different types of back pain can be relieved with Fold and Hold.

(While we will describe various positions depending on the type of back pain, based on Dr. Anderson's analysis, these positions may not cover your case. What do you do? First find a tender spot and then a position of comfort. Once that point is found, adjust your position so that you are folding the body over that tender point. Hold for a minimum of 90 seconds, then gently and slowly release. Then gently stretch that muscle. Remember to think muscular. Look for the muscle in spasm with the goal of putting that muscle to sleep by folding to shorten it and remaining in that hold position for 90 seconds at a minimum, and then gently releasing and finally stretching that muscle to lengthen it and eventually strengthen it.)

General Lower Right- or Left-Sided Back Pain

Typical Symptoms: Standing up straight induces pain; lifting the right thigh or stretching the right thigh backward induces pain; sitting feels better than standing; and the knees propped up while lying on the back offers relief. While the instructions below are designated for the right side, if the pain is on the left side, adapt accordingly.

Potential Cause: Spasm of the ilipsoas muscle, attached to the pelvic bone and to the upper end of the femur (leg bone). Usually this type of back pain is induced after kneeling for a lengthy period of time, then quickly rising. This

247

causes the muscle to go into spasm.

Fold and Hold Techniques:

1. Find the position of comfort. This may be kneeling on the left knee with right knee and thigh close to chest. Here the right iliopsoas muscle is shortened and in relaxed position. Maintain the position for at least 90 seconds, then slowly return to a standing position.

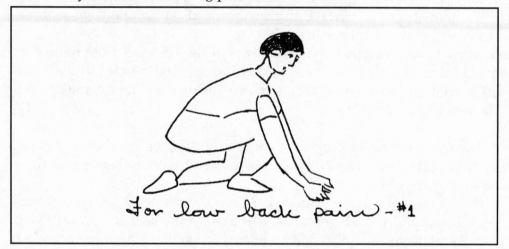

For low back pain - #1

2. Alternatively, sit with the right knee folded up and held under the chin. Hold this position for at least 2 minutes, then slowly return to sitting normally.

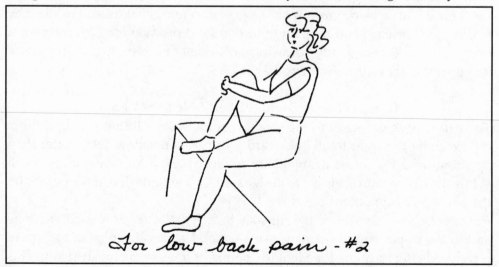

For low back pain - #2

3. If you can remember the position you were in before the spasm developed, try to return to it. If you cannot find it then hold one hand over the tender spot and lie down and bring the right knee to the chest and see if that reduces the pain in the tender spot. If so, move the right foot, thigh, and knee toward the center of the body and bend at the waist a bit to the right. Hold that position for a minimum of 90 seconds and then release slowly.

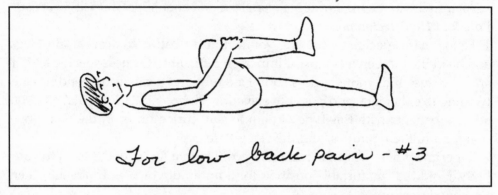

For low back pain - #3

4. An alternative is to locate the tender point—commonly located over or on the outer prominence of the pubic bone. This spot may also be in the groin or the lower abdomen. It is often difficult to touch the tender spot for the pain.

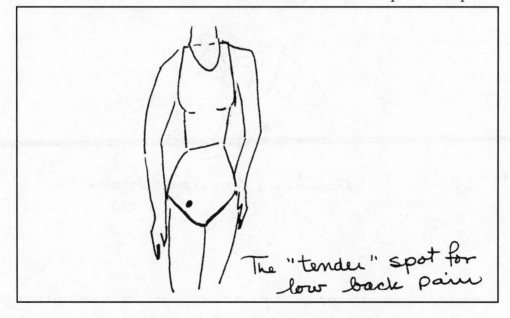

The "tender" spot for low back pain

Low Back Pain That Feels Better When Sitting

Typical Symptoms: With this kind of pain, balling up or tucking the body together relieves pain, but standing, walking, or back-arching makes the pain worse. This is caused by passive stretching of the abdominal and spinal muscles in spasm.

Typical Causes: Sitting in a slouched position, one arises suddenly causing the small muscles in the front of spinal vertebrae and abdominal muscles to spasm.

Fold and Hold Techniques:

1. Follow nature's clue by tucking yourself into a ball with arms around legs and head bent in between knees. It may be difficult to locate a specific tender spot, because the whole back is sore. Fine tune the position by bending and twisting to either side and possibly elevating slightly either leg. Dr. Anderson advises patients with this type of pain to stay curled up or in the Fold position for a full ten minutes, and then slowly release.

2. Experiment here. Find the tucked in position that feels good. Listen to your body. Hold the comfortable position for a minimum of 90 seconds and then slowly release (unfold).

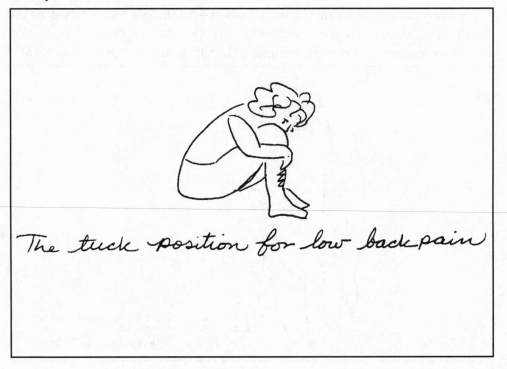

The tuck position for low back pain

Low Back Pain That Feels Better When Standing

Typical Symptoms: Pain is aggravated by sitting or bending forward; bending over a counter or vacuuming aggravates pain. Back pain is improved or relieved when one stands or walks.

Possible Causes: Muscles close to the vertebrae on the back are in spasm generally caused by rapid forward movement. Repetitive lifting may also cause muscles to spasm.

Fold and Hold Techniques:

1. Locate the tender spot. This is normally in the back near the spine. There may be a number of tender spots as several muscles may be in spasm. Once the point is located, stand with the back against a sturdy table or counter, steady yourself with both hands on the table, feet equidistant and anchored, and then slowly arch the back by Folding backwards. Bend backward till the pain in the tender spot diminishes. Hold position for at least 90 seconds and then gently release.

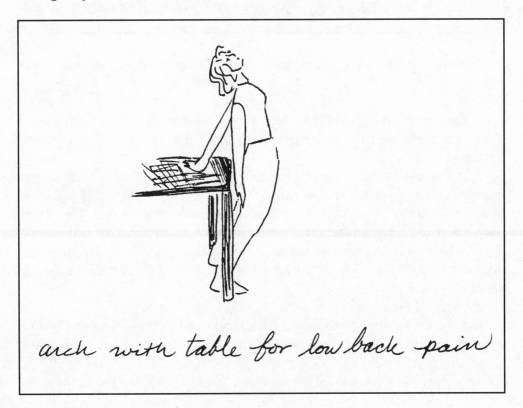

arch with table for low back pain

2. As an alternative, lie on the stomach with both elbows flat on the ground. With the stomach sagging, gently raise yourself upon both elbows and arch the back until the pain in the tender spot diminishes. Then hold for a minimum of 90 seconds and then gently release.

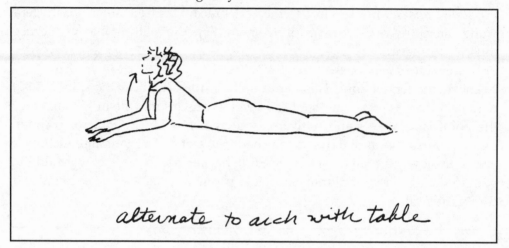

alternate to arch with table

3. Alternatively, lie on your back on a rolled up sheet or towel to arch (fold) the area.

Pain in Right or Left Flank Aggravated by Bending or Twisting

Typical Symptoms: Pain that worsens in the flank area when bending or twisting to the side.

Typical Causes: In this type of pain the quadratus lumborum muscle (the muscle running from the lowest rib in the back to posterior part of pelvis) is in spasm. It usually is caused when pushing something to the left. The object moves and you lunge to the left causing the right quadratus lumborum muscle to dramatically lengthen and then go into spasm. Repetitive loading of the muscle such as lifting and moving a bucket as if you were in a fire brigade can also cause the spasm.

Fold and Hold Techniques:

1. Find the tender spot, in the right flank, and bend to the right and bend or twist backward or forward such that the tender spot pain begins to alleviate. Once you have found the most comfortable position, hold it for 90 seconds and then gently release it. If the tender spot is on the left flank reverse the process.

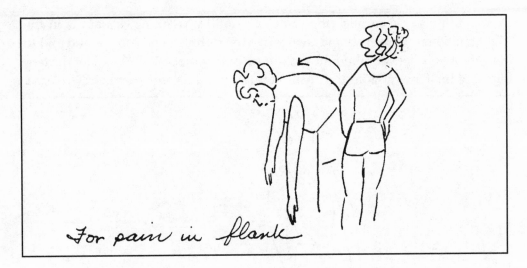

For pain in flank

Tail Bone Pain

Typical Symptoms: Rear end hurts, especially in the tail bone area and it hurts to sit. Tenderness is also felt on either side or directly over tail bone.

Typical Causes: Sudden movements or a fall that causes spasm in the coccygeus muscle, a part of the pelvic diaphragm muscle attached to tail bone.

Fold and Hold Techniques:

1. Lie on the side of the bed on the left side. If the tender spot is to the right side of the tail bone, curl and flex the left leg to a 45 degree angle, then move the right leg behind your body so that it falls to the floor. Adjust the position so that the tender spot starts going away. When the position of maximum comfort is reached, hold the position for 90 seconds. Then gently release. If the pain is on the left side of the tail bone repeat the procedures in the opposite manner.

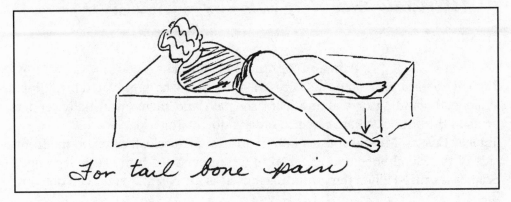

For tail bone pain

2. You can also accomplish the same position by standing. If pain is in the right tail bone, stand erect and then move the right leg and foot behind and to the left of your left leg. Find the maximum position of comfort and let the tender spot melt away. Hold the position for 90 seconds and then gently release.

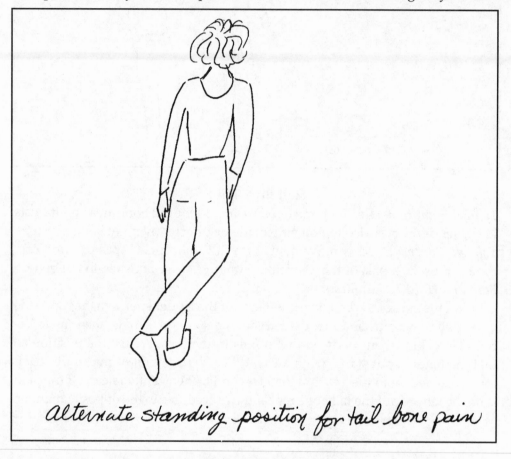

alternate standing position for tail bone pain

Pain and Tightness in Buttocks

Typical Symptoms: Pain or tightness in either buttocks aggravated by sitting. Prolonged standing or walking increases pain and there are usually tender spots in the buttocks. Pain can also radiate down either leg.

Typical Causes: Muscle spasms in the piriformis muscle, located on the front side of the sacral bone and attached to the upper part of the large leg bone. Sciatica is caused when the piriformis muscle is in spasm. If you sleep on your belly with a leg in the frog position and arise suddenly, spasms can result.

Fold and Hold Techniques:

1. Find the tender spot, usually somewhere on the buttocks, generally in the middle. For pain in the right buttock, place the right leg in *a frog position,* on your back or on your stomach, or standing with one leg on a chair. Fine tune or adjust the position so that the tender point is at least 75% relieved. Hold the position for 90 seconds and then release gently. Follow this by stretching the piriformis muscle. Get down on hands and knees in the *cat position.* For pain in the right buttock, move the left leg behind the right leg and stretch downward and to the right. Repeat slowly for a total of three times. For pain in the left buttocks follow the opposite procedure.

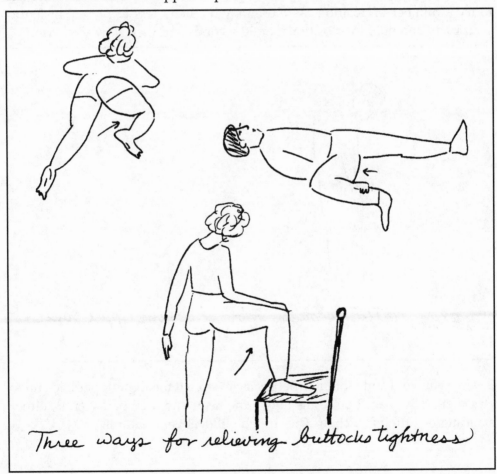

Three ways for relieving buttocks tightness

Upper Back Pain

Typical Symptoms: Standing up induces spasms in the upper back's flexion and extensor muscles.

Typical Causes: Standing or sitting in a slouched position with the head forward. When one rapidly moves from this position flexor and extensor muscles can go into spasm.

Fold and Hold Techniques:

1. Experimentation is the key here. Usually you can locate the tender points in the upper back. Try an *exaggerated slouched position,* see if tender points lessen, then hold for 90 seconds. If that is not successful, arch the back for 90 seconds, and then release slowly. Use whichever is more effective. You also may have to try a number of positions as there may be many tender points. Listen to your body and hold the positions for 90 seconds and then slowly release.

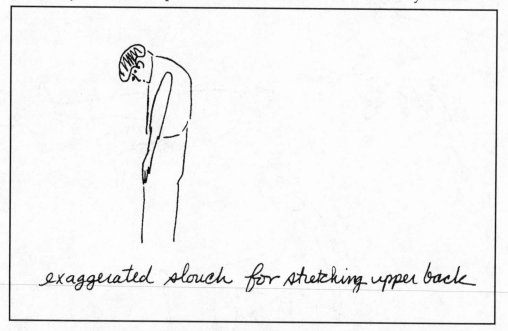

exaggerated slouch for stretching upper back

2. After you Fold and Hold it is necessary to stretch the tight upper back muscles. Generally place both arms above the head and arch back gently, either standing or sitting in a chair. The stretch will feel very natural.

For stretching out upper back

3. Strengthen the upper back muscles by swimming on the floor. Lie on the stomach, slightly raise the right arm out in front of you and at the same time slightly raise the left leg. Then repeat the process with the left arm outstretched and right leg slightly raised. Continue for 5 minutes.

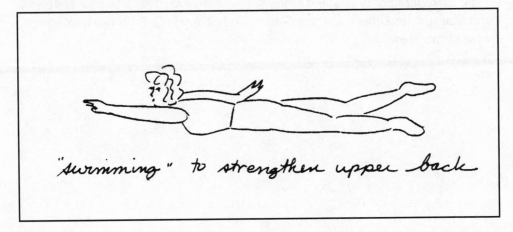

"swimming" to strengthen upper back

Fold and Hold is extremely effective in relieving pain immediately and commencing the healing process.

(We are deeply indebted to Dr. Anderson and Chronimed Publishing for allowing us to share this very effective technique.)

Touch for Health Techniques for Pain Relief

We are very grateful to Dr. John Thie and John Maguire for permitting us to use important materials from their books. We urge you to see a Touch for Health practitioner and learn all you can about this complementary pain relief technique. Practitioner referrals, classes and lay person materials can be obtained from the Kinesiology Institute of America, (800) 501-4878. Touch for Health materials can also be ordered from Devorss Publications at (213) 870-7478. Practitioner referrals can also be obtained from the Touch for Health Association at (800) 466-8342.

The Touch for Health theory and general techniques are fully described in Chapter 22. It is an extremely powerful modality for chronic back pain relief. By taking various physical actions, after muscle testing, including the massaging and holding of various points on the body, muscles can be balanced and re-energized, resulting in pain relief. While muscle testing is an important element of Touch for Health, the following physical methods can be used without testing, and pain relief can be achieved. Each technique will first be generally described and then discussed in relation to specific muscles normally associated with back pain. Please refer to the appropriate charts and illustrations where indicated.

The material here is adapted from *Become Pain Free with Touch for Health* by John Maguire and *Touch For Health* by John F. Thie, D.C. Both books are highly recommended.

The following illustration identifies the major muscle groups in the body and shows the direction of each muscle.

(Reprinted by permission from Touch For Health *by John F. Thie, DC.)*

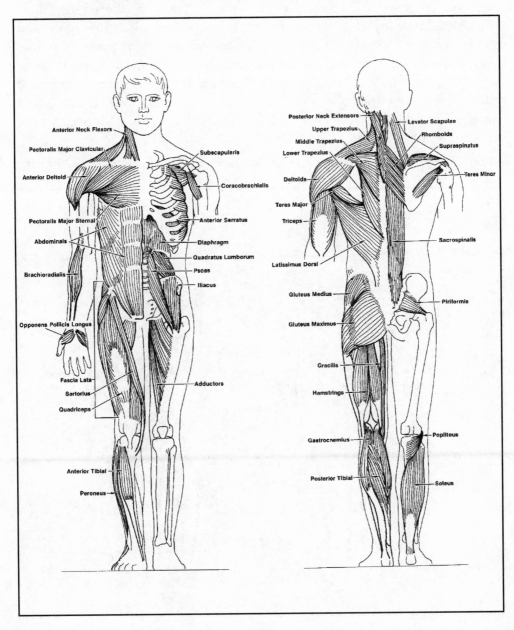

Massage the Neurolymphatic Points: Weak muscles can be reenergized and strengthened by massaging associated neurolymphatic areas consisting of a series of points, which act like circuit breakers in the body. Massaging these points, some of which may be sore, will restore the energy flow, strengthen muscles, unblock energy in a related meridian or organ, and relieve tension and muscular pain. Massage the points or series of points using a deep finger massage technique for approximately 20 seconds. Massage tender or sore points for up to 60 seconds. To enhance the functions of related glands or organs massage the tender points for 30 seconds 2 to 4 times a day. The following chart, "Neurolymphatic Reflexes," illustrates the location of these points.

(Reprinted by permission from Become Pain Free with Touch for Health *by John McGuire)*

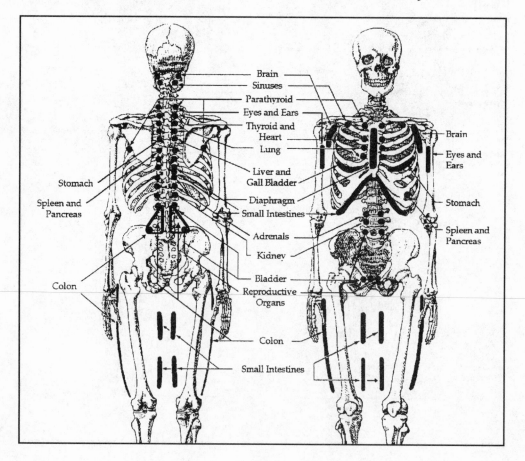

Holding Neurovascular Points: Another technique is to hold neurovascular points, those located on the head, for 20 to 30 seconds. Points related to severe problem areas may be held for up to 5 minutes. This action strengthens the muscles by improving blood circulation to the muscles and related organs, relieves tension and muscular stress, relaxing the body and increasing energy. Hold the points with the pads of the fingers lightly stretching and touching the skin. To enhance the function of related glands or organs hold the related points for 30 seconds 2-4 times per day. Holding all the points once a day as well as the points relating to the muscles associated with chronic back pain is highly recommended. Neurovascular points will be identified in the discussion of each muscle related to back pain and illustrated on the following chart.

(Reprinted by permission from Become Pain Free with Touch for Health *by John McGuire)*

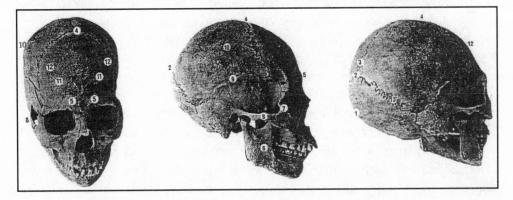

Massaging Muscle While Holding Beginning or End Points of Associated Meridians: Massaging a muscle in the direction of the muscle with one hand while holding the beginning or end point of the associated meridian provides pain relief. Refer to the meridians chart below for their beginning and end points. *Massage Techniques to Weaken Overly Tight Muscles & Release Spasms or Cramps:* 1. Spindle Cell Technique: Much back pain is caused by muscles that are overly tight and shortened or in spasm. To loosen a muscle or release a spasm massage the belly(flat part of muscle) by massaging each end of the muscle's belly inward in the direction of the muscle to the center of the belly. The preferred technique called "tweaken to weaken" involves placing the thumb at one end of the belly and the middle finger at the other end of the muscle's belly and firmly drawing the thumb and middle finger together in the direction of the muscle, or take the 4 fingers at each end of the muscle's belly and rapidly massage inward to the center of the muscle's belly. Repeat the same technique at the other end of the muscle's belly. These techniques tell the brain that the muscle is too short and the brain sends nerve messages to the muscle causing it to relax and loosen.

2. Gogli Tendon Technique: An alternate technique is to massage the ends of a muscle outward towards the origin and insertion points in the direction of a muscle. Apply light pressure pulling towards the origin and insertion points of the muscle whose location is noted under each muscle.

Massage Techniques to Strengthen Weak Muscles:

1. Spindle Cell Technique: Sometimes a muscle is too weak, resulting in an imbalance in an opposite muscle. To strengthen a muscle massage from the center of the belly of a muscle with a firm motion outward to each end of the belly of a muscle. The technique can be accomplished by placing the thumb and middle finger in the center of the belly of a muscle and massaging outward. It is commonly referred to as "lengthen to strengthen". Alternatively one can place the four fingers in the center of the belly and rapidly massage outward towards one end and then the other end of the belly of the muscle. These techniques inform the brain that the muscle is too long. The brain then sends a nerve impulse to the muscle causing it to shorten resulting in strengthening of the muscle.

2. Golgi Tendon Technique: An alternate technique is to place your fingers at the end of a muscle near its origin and insertion points and massage inward towards the belly of the muscle. This technique sends a message to the brain that the muscle does not have enough tension and the brain responds by increasing energy to the muscle resulting in the strengthening of the muscle.

NOTE: These massage techniques *are very important,* as they can be used to strengthen a weak opposing muscle thereby putting a muscle and its opposing muscle into balance, resulting in pain relief. For instance, tight hamstrings causing low back pain, may be loosened by strengthening their opposing muscle group, the quadriceps. If the tight hamstring muscles do not release, you can release them by using the muscle weakening techniques noted above. In the discussion of each muscle related to back pain, the opposing muscle will also be identified.

Massaging Origin and Insertion Points: *The origin of a muscle is on a non-moving bone and the insertion point on a moving bone.* These points are brought closer together when muscles contract. Deeply massaging the origin and insertion points of a muscle for 5-20 seconds tends to wake the muscle up and strengthen it. Origin and insertion points for muscles related to back pain will be noted.

General Meridian Massage: Meridians carry vital energy through the body. Each muscle and organ in the body is associated with a specific meridian. Tracing all the meridians often releases blocked energy resulting in pain reduction or relief. Using an open-palmed flat hand, trace the direction of the meridian from beginning to end. Use both hands to trace the right and left sides simultaneously. *You do not have to touch the body. Stroking two inches above the skin is generally ideal.* The following chart illustrates the meridians, and the written directions below specify how each is to be massaged.

(Reprinted by permission from Become Pain Free with Touch for Health *by John McGuire)*

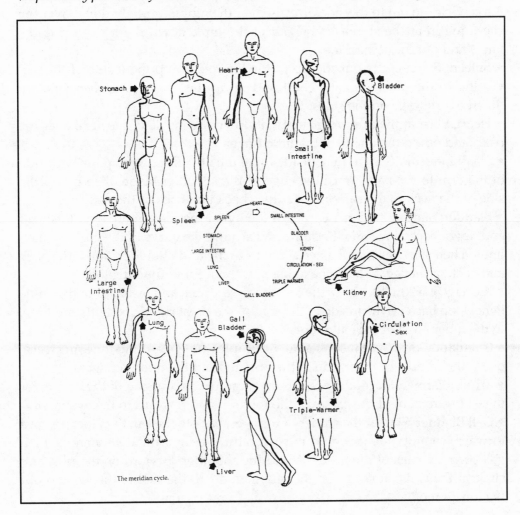

The meridian cycle.

Commence the massage by tracing the central and governing meridians and then proceed with the stomach meridian and follow around the circle in the order noted on the chart. The cycle can be repeated. (We suggest you tape record these directions for play-back to direct you while massaging the meridians.)

• Central: Start at the pubic bone, go up the midline to the bottom of the lip.

• Governing: Start at the tailbone, go up the spine, over the top of the head and over the nose to the upper lip.

• Stomach: Start under the pupil of the eye, to straight down the jaw, circle up around the face to the frontal eminences, drop straight down over the eye to the clavicle, go out to the side directly over the nipple, straight down over the chest, jog in at the stomach and out at the hips, down the leg (outside the knee) and out the second toe.

• Spleen: Start on the outside tip of the big toe, go up the inside of the leg, veering to the outside of the chest and up to the arm crease, then halfway down the rib cage on the sides.

• Heart: Start at the armpit, go straight down the inside of the arm, over the palm and out to the inside of the little finger.

• Small Intestine: Start at the outside tip of the little finger, go up the back side of the arm to the back, trace the edge of the shoulder blade, then go up the side of the neck to the earlobe, over the cheek and back to the ear.

• Bladder: Start at the inner corner of the top of the eyes, go up over the head and down back alongside the spine and around the curve of the gluteus maximus. Then start again at the neck, go out to the mid-shoulder, down the back and back of the leg, behind the ankle bone and out to the little toe.

• Kidney: Start on the ball of the foot, go up the arch and just back of the ankle bone, loop back on the inside of the leg, up the chest right next to the midline, to the inner edge of the collar bone.

• Circulation-Sex: Start just outside the nipples and go around the arm crease, down the middle of the inside of the arm and out the middle finger.

• Triple Warmer: Start at the third finger, go up the outside of the arm, over the elbow, to behind the ear, over the top of it and forward to the eyebrow.

• Gall Bladder: Start at the corner of the eyes, back to the ear, then loop up and forward, coming down behind the ear, return to the frontal eminences, then go down the back of the head, behind the shoulder, forward on the ribs, half circle at the waist, forward on the hip, then down the side of the leg and out the fourth toe.

• Liver: Start on the inside of the big toes, forward on the edge of the ribs about halfway towards the center.

• Lung: Start on the upper chest just inside the top of the arm, down the outside of the arm through the palm to the thumb.

• Large Intestine: Start from the top of the index finger, go up the outside, top of the arm, over the shoulder, to the front of the neck to the corner of the mouth, under the base of the nose ending next to the flare of the nose on the opposite side.

Flushing A Meridian: Locate the meridian that is closest to the pain site. With quick light movements trace that meridian from beginning to end to beginning about 5 times. Then trace the meridian from beginning to end and then from end to the beginning. Try to determine which stroking direction gave you the most pain relief. Then stroke the meridian in the pain relieving direction until the pain lessens, or a maximum of 50 times.

Holding the Painful Area While Massaging the Related Meridian: Lightly holding the area of pain, while at the same time massaging the associated meridian slowly from the beginning of the meridian to its end with the index and middle fingers in a firm manner will often relieve pain. In the event two finger massage reveals additional pain points along the way, massage those additional points firmly until the pain is eliminated.

Fascia Release Technique: Muscles are surrounded by a fascial sheath. Ideally the muscle and its fascial sheath should be the same length and function as a unit. The fascia should move smoothly as muscles relax and contract. Fascia which are shorter than the muscle can cause friction and tension resulting in pain and limitation of range of motion. To lengthen the fascia place a little oil or lotion on the muscle and massage with firm pressure in the direction of the muscle towards the heart. Massage the muscle 3-4 times.

Feathering A Muscle: A cramping muscle can be released through the feathering technique. Rub the sore muscle with the fingers in a brisk manner with a feathery touch. Increase the pressure and rub briskly if pain is not at first relieved. Stretching the muscle while feathering it is also helpful.

How To Use the Pain Relief Techniques

If you are in pain, or you detect an area of tightness in the back or associated muscles, locate that area on the muscle chart in order to find the appropriate muscle or opposing muscle to work on. Generally pain and tightness result from muscle imbalances. The tight and painful muscle is in spasm or contracted because the opposing muscle is weak. First, use the strengthening techniques to bring the opposing muscle into balance so that the tight and painful muscle will loosen. If that does not fully loosen the tight muscle, then use weakening techniques on the tight muscle. Massage the neurolymphatic and neurovascular holding points to balance the original tight muscle and the original weak muscle. Massage the origin and holding points of the tight and opposing muscles. If pain is still present, then massage the painful muscle in the direction of the muscle while holding the beginning and end points of the related meridian. Then hold the painful area while massaging along the related meridian giving special attention to sore points. If pain is still present, then use myofascial release and the feathering technique. Finally, flush the meridian associated with the painful muscle and finish up with a general meridian massage. This comprehensive approach should lead to pain reduction or elimination.

Touch for Health Techniques For Muscles Associated with Back Pain

Using the above Touch for Health techniques on the following specific muscles associated with back pain should reduce or eliminate pain, while at the same time balance key muscles. These muscles include: hamstrings, adductors, fascia lata, quadriceps, psoas, piriformis, gluteus maximus, gluteus medius, sacrospinalis, lattisimus dorsi and quadratus lumborum. *Refer to the chart of muscles for the location and direction of each muscle.* Also, within each muscle's discussion, refer to *the neurolymphatic reflexes chart* and the *neurovascular holding points chart* where indicated. To help you understand each muscle's function relative to the back, its action will be described.

Experimentation will be in order, but the techniques are highly effective for pain relief. Note down each technique that results in pain relief and use the helpful ones daily. The phrase "uncontract muscles on your pain management contract" also refers to using Touch for Health techniques.

Piriformis Muscle:
1. Action and Relevance to Back Pain: The piriformis muscle rotates the hip laterally and abducts the flexed thigh at the hip. An improperly balanced and weakened piriformis muscle can cause significant back and leg pain.
2. Meridian: Circulation Sex, on each side of the body. See circulation sex on meridian chart and tracing directions.

3. Neurolymphatic Holding Points: (See chart above.)

   a. Front of Body: The entire length of the pubic bone.

   b. Back of Body: Prominent knobs of the hip bones.

4. Neurovascular Holding Points: Ridge between the ear and top of the head. Point 10 on chart of neurovascular holding points.

5. Opposing Muscles: Gracilis, semitendinosus, semi-membrarosus, and adductors.

6. Origin: Inner surface of sacral and hip bones

7. Insertion: Inner surface of sacral and hip bones.

Psoas Muscle:

1. Action and Relevance to Back Pain: The psoas muscle flexes the thigh at the hip. When the thigh is flexed, the psoas muscle pulls on the vertebrae and flexes the spine and pelvis on the thigh. An unbalanced psoas muscle is a major cause of back and leg pain in view of its size and location in the hip and its attachment to the back's vertebrae.

2. Meridian: Kidney, on each side of the body. See kidney meridian on meridian chart and tracing directions.

3. Neurolymphatic Holding Points: See chart.

   a. Front of Body: One inch from side of navel and one inch above navel.

   b. Back: One inch to each side of the spine between thoracic vertebrae 12 and lumbar vertebrae 12, just below level of the last ribs.

4. Neurovascular Holding Points: The prominent bump in the back of the head near the base of the skull. Point 1 on chart of neurovascular holding points.

5. Opposing Muscles: Hamstring and opposite psoas.

6. Origin: Along the spine from T 12, the level of the last rib, and all the lumbar vertebrae.

7. Insertion: Inside of the upper part of the thigh bone, about level with the pubic bone.

Hamstring Muscle:

1. Action and Relevance to Back Pain: There are medial and lateral hamstring muscles on the back of the thighs. These muscles rotate and flex the leg at the knee as well as extend, adduct, and rotate the thigh at the hip. Tight hamstring muscles are a major cause of back pain as they pull down on the muscles in the buttocks as well as the lower and mid-back.

2. Meridian: Large Intestines, on each side of the body. See large intestines on the meridian chart and tracing directions.

3. Neurolymphatic Holding Points: See chart.

    a. Front of Body: Points inside of the upper thighs.

    b. Back of Body: Most prominent knobs on hip bones at lumbar vertebrae 5.

4. Neurovascular Holding Points: See point 2 on the chart. The soft spot on the back of the head.

5. Opposing Muscles: Quadriceps in relation to the rotating of the knee the biceps femoris(medial). Quadriceps in relation to hip and knee, and in rotation of the knee, the gracilis, semitendinosus, semimembranousis(lateral).

6. Origin: On the back, the lowest part of the hip bone upon which one sits on both sides.

7. Insertion: Top of the bones of the lower leg, inside back and outside of the leg, just below the knee.

Tensor Fascia Lata Muscle:

1. Action and Relevance to Back Pain: The tensor fascia lata muscles are located on the outside of each thigh. These muscles are responsible for flexion, abduction and medial rotation at the hip. Tight tensor fascia lata muscles are also a major cause of back pain as they pull down on the buttocks and lower back.

2. Meridian: Large Intestine, on each side of the body. See large intestine on the meridian chart and tracing directions.

3. Neurolymphatic Holding Points: See chart.

    a. Front of Body: Top of the thigh bone to 1 inch below the outside of both legs.

    b. Back of Body: The triangular area from lumbar vertebrae 2 and 4 to the highest part of the hip bones.

4. Neurovascular Holding Points: See point 10 on the chart. The ridge between the ear and top of the head.

5. Opposing Muscles: Adductors

6. Origin: Outer edge of the hip bone, toward the front.

7. Insertion: Just below the knee on the outside of the leg.

Adductor Muscle:

1. Action and Relevance to Back Pain: These muscles, on both sides of the inner thighs, hold the thigh in and flex it in and outward. Weakness of these muscles can make the pelvis tilt downward. Weak adductors, the opposing muscles of tensor fascia lata, can result in tight tensor fascia lata that pull on muscles in the hips and lower back. They can also result in tight muscles in the buttocks if they are weak.

2. Meridian: Circulation- Sex, on each side of the body. See circulation sex on meridian chart and tracing directions.

3. Neurolymphatic Holding Points: See chart.

   a. Front of Body: Behind the nipple on the chest wall, between 4th and-5th ribs.

   b. Back of Body: Just below the points of the shoulder blades, between the 8th and 9th ribs.

4. Neurovascular Holding Points: Point 10 on the chart. The ridge between the ear and top of the head and on the sides at the back of the skull.

5. Opposing Muscles: Tensor fascia lata, gluteus maximus and sartorius.

6. Origin: Front of the pubic bones.

7. Insertion: Front of the thigh bone just below the hip to the inside of the knee and just below the knee on the inside of the shin bone.

Quadricep Muscle:

1. Action and Relevance to Back Pain: These muscles are responsible for straightening the knee and flexing the hip. Weak quadriceps can result in a muscle imbalance in the hamstrings resulting in tight hamstrings that pull on the muscles of the buttocks and back.

2. Meridian: Small Intestines, on each side of the body. See small intestine on meridian chart and tracing directions.

3. Neurolymphatic Holding Points.

   a. Front of Body: A series of points between the 8th, 9th, 10th and 11th ribs near the cartilage, along the curve at the bottom of the front of the rib cage.

   b. Back of Body: Between thoracic vertebrae 8,9,10, 11 and 12, one inch to each side of the spine.

4. Neurovascular Holding Points: Point 10 on the neurovascular holding point chart. The ridge between the ear and top of the head.

5. Origin: Upper portion of the thigh bone and side of the hip bone.

6. Insertion: On the shin bone just below the knee cap.

Gluteus Maximus Muscle:

1. Action and Relevance to Back Pain: This large muscle is responsible for stabilizing the low back and extends the thigh and pulls the leg in. A weak gluteus maximus can result in a destabilized back resulting in pain.

2. Meridian: Circulation Sex on each side of the body. See circulation sex on the meridian chart and tracing directions.

3. Neurolymphatic Holding Points: See chart.

   a. Front of Body: From the top of the thigh bone down to just above the knees on the outside of the legs.

    b. Back of the Body: The most prominent knob on the hip bones at the level of the 5th lumbar vertebrae.

4. Neurovascular Holding Points: Point 13 on the chart. On the left side at the back of the skull.

5. Opposing Muscles: Adductors, piriformis and neck muscles.

6. Origin: Back of the hip bones across the surface of the sacrum.

7. Insertion: Top, back of the thigh bone, down about 3 inches.

Gluteus Medius Muscle:

1. Action and Relevance to Back Pain: The gluteus medius muscle pulls the thigh out and rotates the leg. If there is weakness in this muscle back pain may result because of tight psoas or fascia lata muscles.

2. Meridian: Circulation-Sex, on each side of the body. See circulation sex on meridian chart and tracing directions.

3. Neurolymphatic Holding Points: See chart above.

    a. Front of Body: A series of points across the upper edge of the pubic bone.

    b. Back of Body: Most prominent knob on the hip bone at level of lumbar vertebrae 5.

4. Neurovascular Holding Points: Point 10 on the chart. The ridge between the ear and top of the head.

5. Opposing Muscles: Psoas and fascia lata.

6. Origin: Outer surface of the hip bones.

7. Insertion: Top of the thigh bone at the side.

Sascrospinalis Muscle:

1. Action and Relevance to Back Pain. These muscles are the major muscles along the back bone. They are responsible for the extension, flexion and lateral movement of the vertebrae column. If these muscles are out of balance they can be the cause of significant pain along the spine.

2. Meridian: Bladder, on each side of the body. See bladder on the meridian chart and tracing directions.

3. Neurolymphatic Holding Points.

    a. Front of Body: The series of points along the pubic bone and the two points on each side of the naval.

    b. Back of Body: About 1.5 inches from the spine at lumbar vertebrae 2 level with the lowest part of the rib cage.

4. Neurovascular Holding Points: Point 11 on the chart. Between the eyebrows

and hairline on the forehead.

5. Opposing Muscles: Abdominal muscles and the right sacrospinalis opposes the left sacrospinalis and vice versa.

6. Origin: Muscles arising from the sacrum running through hip bones to the base of the skull. Shorter fibers run from one vertebrae to the next and longer fibers run the whole length of the back.

7. Insertion: See discussion under origin.

Abdominal Muscle:

1. Action and Relevance to Back Pain: There are two sets of abdominal muscles: the rectus abdominis running in the center of the belly and two transverse abdominal muscles running on each side of the rectus abdominus muscle. These muscles are responsible for keeping the organs in place, keeping the pelvis up and compressing the abdomen. Weak abdominal muscles can result in a beer belly. More importantly weak abdominal muscles result in very tight sacrospinalis muscles which lead to back pain.

2. Meridian: Small Intestines, on each side of the body. See small intestines on the meridian chart and tracing directions.

3. Neurolymphatic Holding Points: See chart.

    a. Front of Body: Inside of the thighs on three areas. These bands of points are slightly forward and back.

    b. Back of Body: The most prominent knob on the hip bones at the level of lumbar vertebrae 5 and on the back inside of thighs from sitting bones to $1/3$ down the back of thigh.

    c. Skull Bones: Place hands at top of skull with fingers spread along the middle part of skull and pull the scalp apart about 5 times with heavy pressure.

4. Neurovascular Holding Points: Point 10 on the neurovascular holding points chart. The prominent ridge between the ear and the top of the head.

5. Opposing Muscles: Sacrospinalis, quadriceps, hamstrings, psoas, latissimus dorsi, pectorals, gluteus medius and maximus.

6. Origin: For transverse muscles, in the inner surfaces of the lower six ribs, diaphragm and back of the hips. For rectus, on the surface of the lower 8 ribs.

7. Insertion: Along the abdomen from the sternum to the pubic bone, for the transverse muscles. For the rectus muscles on the upper edges of the hip and pubic bones.

Quadratus Lumborum Muscle:

1. Action and Relevance to Back Pain: This muscle is responsible for sideways flexion of the vertebral column. It is a major stabilizing muscle of the lower

back. Weakness of this muscle can result in a destabilized back.

2. Meridian: Large Intestines, on each side of the body. See large intestine on the meridian chart and tracing directions.

3. Neurolymphatic Holding Points.

    a. Front of Body: On the top of the iliac crest and a series of points in a band on the inside top half of the thigh to the inside of the quadriceps muscles.

    b. Back of Body: A series of points on the inward part of the upper thighs.

4. Neurovascular Holding Points: Point 10 on the chart. At the ridge between the ear and top of the head.

5. Opposing Muscles: One side opposes the other and the opposite sacrospinalis muscle.

6. Origin: Along the top rear of the iliac crest and along the iliolumbar ligament.

7. Insertion: Between the edge of the 12th rib and along the transverse process of the upper 4 lumbar vertebrae.

Latisimus Dorsi Muscle:

1. Action and Relevance to Back Pain: These major muscles in the back hold the shoulders down and keep the back straight. A weakness in these muscles will tend to destabilize the back.

2. Meridian: Spleen, on each side of the body. See spleen on the meridian chart and tracing directions.

3. Neurolymphatic Holding Points.

    a. Front of Body: Between the 7th and 8th ribs near the cartilage, usually on the left. There can be a depression there.

    b. Back of Body: Between the 7th and 8th thoracic vertebrae about one inch to each side of the spine.

4. Neurovascular Holding Points: Point 3 on the chart. On the parietal bone just above and behind the ear.

5. Opposing Muscles: Pectorals and deltoids.

6. Origin: Along the length of the spine from the 6th thoracic vertebra between the lower part of the shoulder blades, down to the level of the hips to the top of the hip bones in the back.

7. Insertion: Inside of the arm just below the shoulder.

CHAPTER 27

NUTRITIONAL ASPECTS OF PAIN RELIEF: VITAMINS, MINERALS, AMINO ACIDS, HERBS, AND DIET

THIS CHAPTER DEALS WITH DIETARY SUPPLEMENTS that can help relieve pain and with basic dietary considerations for chronic pain patients. We suggest various supplements and foods that can greatly enhance the physical and mental means of pain relief already presented.

The Vitamins

Vitamins play a vital role in the life process by regulating the body's metabolism and assisting the biochemical process that releases energy from digested food. Vitamins are classified into water soluble vitamins that cannot be stored in the body and are excreted within 1 to 4 days (B complex and C), and fat soluble vitamins that are stored in the body's fatty tissue (Vitamins A D, E, and K). The recommended dosages herein are principally derived from *Prescription for Nutritional Healing* by Balch and Balch, a good compendium of research on vitamins, and also from *Life Without Pain* by Dr. Richard M. Linchitz (where noted).

Chronic back pain sufferers may have vitamin and mineral deficiencies due to prolonged stress and depression. Vitamins and minerals can relieve pain and soothe anxiety. In our discussion we will note the suggested dosage and purpose of the vitamin or mineral. *If no dosage is indicated, follow the dosage instructions on the bottle.* Amino acids also play a very significant role in pain relief.

Please note: Do not exceed dosages recommended here and do not fall into the trap of "if this much makes me feel good, a lot more will make me feel great." Greater than recommended dosages can be harmful. Check with your physician before taking any of the vitamins, minerals, or supplements suggested in this chapter.

Vitamin C (Ascorbic Acid)

Purpose: Vitamin C has been called a "wonder drug," because it has been used in the healing of many different ailments. Relative to chronic pain, vitamin C assists in tissue repair and reduces tension in the back area.

Dosage: 3,000-5,000 milligrams daily.

Food Source: Citrus foods; strawberries; melons; potatoes; dark green vegetables; green peppers; and tomatoes.

Vitamin B6

Purpose: Vitamin B6 is used to repair injured back muscles, and assists in energy production and red blood cell formation.

Dosage: 100 milligrams daily

Food Source: Whole grain bread (not enriched); green leafy vegetables; cereal and bread; avocados; liver; bananas; green beans; fish; poultry; meats; and nuts.

Vitamin B Complex Formula

Purpose: A vitamin B complex formula is most useful in relieving stress and repairing muscle tissue.

Dosage: One time daily in doses noted on bottle.

Food Source: Vitamin B1 (pork, liver, oysters, whole grain bread, pasta, peas, lima bean, and wheat germ); Vitamin B2 (liver, eggs, dark green vegetables, whole grain bread, enriched cereals, pasta, mushrooms, dried peas and beans); Vitamin B3 (liver, poultry, meat, tuna, eggs, nuts, whole grain and enriched cereals, dried peas and beans);

Vitamin B6 (see above); Vitamin B12 (see below).

Vitamin B12

Purpose: Assists in calcium absorption, proper functioning of nervous system and building genetic material.

Dosage: 2,000 micrograms daily in sublingual form.

Food Source: Liver; kidneys; meat; fish; eggs; milk; and oysters.

Vitamin A

Purpose: Critical to proper metabolism of muscle, and helps build supple skin, clear eyes, and strong teeth.

Dosage: 25,000 I.U. daily. Note: Overdoses of this vitamin can be toxic.

Food Source: Liver; cream cheese; eggs; butter; milk; orange and dark green vegetables, papaya, cantaloupe.

Vitamin E

Purpose: Critical to muscles and bones, and red blood cell formation.

Dosage: 400-800 I.U. daily.
Food Source: Vegetable oils; margarine; whole grain cereals and bread; liver; dried beans; and leafy green vegetables

The Minerals

Minerals come from the earth and are passed to humans in the food chain in various plant and animal food sources. In describing the need for minerals, the authors of *Prescription for Nutritional Healing* state that minerals "...are needed for the proper composition of the body fluids, the formation of blood and bone, and the maintenance of healthy nerve function." The recommended minerals and their dosages are principally derived from that book. Minerals are divided into two categories: Major minerals, those needed in grams and less; and trace minerals, those needed in tiny amounts, usually measured in millionths of a gram.

Zinc

Purpose: Valuable in muscle and bone metabolism.
Dosage: 50 milligrams daily.
Food Source: Distributed in vegetables.

Boron

Purpose: Improves uptake of calcium, needed for muscle and bone repair.
Dosage: 3 milligrams daily

Manganese Glutenate

Purpose: An aid to healing muscle tissue in the neck and back.
Dosage: 2-5 milligrams daily

Calcium

Purpose: Strengthens bones, essential to muscle function.
Dosage: 1,500-2,000 milligrams daily
Food Source: Milk products; fish; eggs; beans; fruits; vegetables; whole grains.

Magnesium

Purpose: Strengthens bones, affects muscle contraction, and nerve conduction.
Dosage: 400 milligrams of chelated magnesium daily.
Food Source: Nuts; seafood; whole grains and green, leafy vegetables.

Amino Acids

Amino acids are the "building blocks"of protein. Protein is present in, and provides the structure for, every living organism. "Protein substances make up the muscles, ligaments, tendons, organs, glands, and body fluids…and are essential for the growth of bones." Amino acids play a role in the receiving and sending of messages to the brain. See *Prescriptions for Nutritional Healing.*

DLPA

One amino acid, DLPA, has proved very effective in the relief of pain and is available at your local health food store. In *Life Without Pain*, Dr. Linchitz tells us that DLPA contains the "raw material" for two important "depression fighting" neurotransmitters that relieve depression and make us feel good.
Purpose: Relieves pain and depression, helps with bone tissue repair.
Dosage: Start with 500 milligrams four times a day, with meals and before bedtime. If there is no improvement, add 500 mgs. four times a day, and continue until the pain and depression symptoms show marked improvement. Then reduce the intake of DLPA by 500 mgs. a day. If symptoms re-appear, go *back* to the previous day's dosage. Be sure you are taking ample dosages of Vitamin C and B 6. This is a high dosage, but Dr. Linchitz feels that chronic pain sufferers need more than the average person. *Discuss this dosage with your physician before taking.* Also watch for the symptoms of overdose: insomnia, irritability, possibly belligerence. Cut back if you experience these side effects.
Caution: DLPA should not be taken by those with high blood pressure, who are diabetic, or pregnant.
Food Source: Peanuts; almonds; turkey; liver; chicken; veal; lamb; halibut; cheddar cheese and cottage cheese.

L-Tryptophan

Purpose: L-Tryptophan is a natural amino acid. Increased levels of this amino acid raise serotonin levels in the brain, thus increasing your tolerance for pain as well as prolonging sleep, calming nerves, and curbing the appetite.

Dosage: Studies have shown that an adult needs only 3 milligrams of this amino acid per day. While the FDA has recalled L-Tryptophan supplements because they are associated with a blood disease, eating various foods rich in this amino acid in moderate amounts does not seem to be a problem.

Food Source: Four ounces of veal, lean beef, chicken, fish, eight ounces of nonfat milk, one ounce of cheese, 1 cup of green vegetables, $^1/_2$ cup of pasta, 1 tortilla, or one serving of fruit will supply the daily needed doses of this amino acid.

Tyrosine

Purpose: Like DLPA, tyrosine is an amino acid that converts to depression-fighting neurotransmitters.

Dosage: Healthy amounts of tyrosine can be easily obtained in foods, so generally supplements are not recommended.

Food Source: $^1/_2$ cup peanuts, 6 tablespoons of peanut butter, 2 large eggs, 3 ounces of chicken, liver, veal, lamb, ham, or halibut provide sufficient tyrosine. (from *Life Without Pain*).

L-Lysine and L-Arginine

Purpose: To relieve morning stiffness. Highly effective.

Dosage: 500 mg. of each daily, generally in the evening. But try taking it at other times of the day if taking it in the evening does not relieve stiffness the next morning.

The Herbs

Healers of many cultures the world over have long relied on the therapeutic properties in herbs to treat virtually every ailment known to man. Herbs can deaden pain and heal damaged tissues, and they have anti-spasmodic and anti-inflammatory properties. Herbs come in capsules, liquid, or their natural form as powder and roots. Chronic back pain and its accompanying anxiety, nervousness, and depression have successfully been treated with these natural botanical medicines. We have divided the herbs into two categories: those for pain relief and rebuilding tissues, and those for treating anxiety and nervousness. Most of the herbs are available at health food stores. Many recommendations noted here also come from *Prescription for Nutritional Healing*.

HERBS FOR PAIN RELIEF AND REBUILDING TISSUE

White Willow
Purpose: White willow is a pain reliever, similar to aspirin. It has anti-inflammatory, anti-rheumatic, antiseptic and analgesic properties. It is highly effective for muscle pains.
Dosage: Administer dosages of 5 ml. fluid extract three times a day. Also available in capsule form with other herbs. Follow directions on label.

Comfrey
Purpose: Comfrey plays a critical role because of its main ingredient allatonin for cartilage, bone and muscle cell growth
Dosage: As a cream, rub it on affected area as frequently as required.

Skullcap
Purpose: Used primarily as an antispasmodic and to calm nerves.
Dosage: Mix 5 ml. lemon balm and 45 ml. skullcap tincture and use up to four 5 ml. doses a day to calm nerves and serve as an antispasmodic. Also available in capsule form with other herbs; follow directions on label.

Devils Claw
Purpose: Has strong anti-inflammatory properties as well as analgesic and sedative properties.
Dosage: Take 1 to 3 grams in powder form a day by capsule in the acute phases, then taper back to 15 ml. of tincture a day.

Feverfew
Purpose: Used traditionally as an anti-inflammatory. It is a strong analgesic and blood vessel dilator. Has been reported to have very good success with back pain and soreness.
Dosage: Take in capsule form and follow directions on the label.

Combination Herbal Capsules
Purpose: Many health food stores sell combination capsules containing many of the ingredients noted above in mixed capsule form. A typical arthritis or muscle painrelieving capsule will contain such items as white willow bark,

hops, devils claw and feverfew.
Dosage: Follow the directions on the label.

HERBS TO COMBAT NERVOUSNESS, ANXIETY, AND DEPRESSION

Valerian
Purpose: Valerian is a very powerful natural tranquilizer without any of the side or habit forming effects of medicinal tranquilizers. It also lowers blood pressure and serves as an antispasmodic
Dosage: Usually taken in capsule form; follow directions on the bottle. Due to its strength, you may want to experiment with half a capsule to see effects. 445 mg. capsules are very strong. It is also available in liquid form. Can also be taken as a tea, generally before bed time

Skullcap
Purpose: A strong relaxant, effective for treating nervousness.
Dosage: Take as a powered herb in capsule form. Follow directions on the label, though you may want to consider modifying the dose because of its strong effects.

Chamomile
Purpose: Has strong sedative and antispasmodic properties.
Dosage: Chamomile tea is widely available, and should be used whenever you feel anxious. Drinking 5 cups of chamomile tea a day has proven effective in the relief of back pain. Also available in ointment form.

Borage
Purpose: Effective in treatment of anxiety and depression as well as being anti-rheumatic.
Dosage: For relief of depression and anxiety, pulp the leaves and drink 10 ml. of juice three times a day. It tends to stimulate the adrenal glands, so tailor the dosage.

Combination Herbal Capsules
Many health food stores also have combination capsules that contain the above noted ingredients as well as others that have proved effective in treat-

ing anxiety, depression, nervousness, panic attacks, and other psychological effects of chronic back pain. Follow instructions on label.

Consulting an Herbalist

In many states, especially in the Western United States, herbalists, including Chinese herbalists, can be consulted for specific herbal prescriptions. Herbs may be better if you are having significant side effects from Western medicines. Chinese herbalists will usually prescribe a number of different herbs that are normally boiled into a tea. There are also many books on herbal healing. Check with the public library or local health food store, which may also have a list of herbalists in your area.

Weight Management and Good Nutrition

Extra weight, especially in the abdomen, can cause or significantly increase chronic back pain levels. Picture a man whose big Santa-like belly pulls the back and spine forward. In order for the body to be balanced with this forward thrust, the back muscles must work hard to compensate, increasing tension levels. If your back is sore, consider the pressures and increased pain levels extra abdominal weight may be causing. If you have significant weight in the belly, losing weight should reduce pressure on the back and therefore, reduce pain. Most Americans are overweight to some degree, and so for most people, weight loss should be part of a back pain management program. Having perhaps been in chronic pain for some months, you may have been less physically active and put on weight as a result, and this, of course does not help the back. Good nutrition also contributes to strong bones and muscles, making a stronger, healthier back.

How To Lose Weight and Keep it Off

Losing weight is a passion in our country. Literally billions of dollars and countless hours are spent finding an easy way to lose weight. But there really is no easy way. Effective long-term weight loss involves a steady, committed program, in which you lose a few pounds a week, eating a healthy, low-fat diet with lots of exercise. It really is about calories and exercise, as opposed to magic diets, pills, or liquid or pre-packaged meals. You can lose weight without spending a fortune by following a low-fat, high-fiber diet, along with a regular exercise program. Consult your physician or nutritionist for appropriate diet suggestions

Holistic Dietary Guidelines

Even if you are not overweight, following the guidelines below can increase general health and well-being, and that, of course, will enhance a pain management program.

• Eat a balanced diet, keeping processed foods to a minimum.

• Eliminate or significantly reduce foods high in fat, sugar and salt.

• Eliminate or keep red meat to a minimum (no more than once a week)

• Emphasize fiber and fresh fruit in the diet.

• Significantly reduce or eliminate dairy products as they congest the system.

• Eliminate or drastically reduce the intake of caffeine.

• Avoid foods that may take away from vital energy including: melted cheese, milk products, chocolate, coffee, black tea, alcohol, fried foods, beef, pork, hydrogenated or partially hydrogenated oils, or heavily processed food containing preservatives, artificial flavorings and colors.

• Chew food thoroughly and eat slowly.

• Remain upright while eating and digesting.

• Do not drink with meals, though a small glass of wine is appropriate.

• As fruit is difficult to digest, do not eat it with a meal.

• For an energy pickup, eat fruit at mid-morning and mid-afternoon.

• Eat foods rich in vitamin C such as citrus fruit, melons, sprouts, and broccoli.

• Eat foods rich in magnesium such as bell peppers, lettuce, nuts, and seafood.

• Eat foods rich in potassium such as beans, bananas, whole grains.

• Include plenty of complex carbohydrates in the diet: whole, non-animal source foods, such as fresh fruits and vegetables, and unprocessed grains, such as whole wheat and brown rice. Avoid or significantly limit white flour products such as pastries, white bread, and pasta.

• Drink 10 glasses of water a day. Water is nature's most critical nutrient in the body as it helps remove waste products and toxins. *Back pain has een linked to a shortage of water in the body.*

• An excellent substitute for coffee is "sweet" water. Mix three parts water with one part apple juice. This mixture, taken throughout the day, will keep you hydrated, awake, and focused without any of the side effects of caffeine.

• Keep a food diary by day and meal indicating time, foods eaten, energy level, emotional level and pain levels. In this manner you can track the foods that assist in reducing pain levels and anxiety.

CHAPTER 28

RECOMMENDED PAIN MANAGEMENT PROGRAMS

Introduction

WE HAVE NOW REACHED THE MOST IMPORTANT CHAPTER, where we suggest goals, activities, and the most effective pain management/pain control techniques. There are three recommended programs:

• Long Form—designed for those who have time and energy to meet its demands and challenges.

• Short Form—designed for those who cannot devote the time needed to carry out the long form program.

• Design-Your-Own—contains the minimum basic requirements for any back pain management program. Goal activities in areas of social, recreational, vocational, and pain flare-ups need to be established.

Goal setting and accomplishment are the foundation of each program. Each goal activity will be discussed briefly, and a weekly frequency for each activity will be recommended. Goals and goal activities will be noted on sample pain management contracts for each of the three programs. Copy the appropriate form so you can use it in checking off activities as you complete them. The term "optional" beside a goal activity means it is not mandatory, but is something that will enhance the effectiveness of a program.

These programs are designed to distract you from pain; to teach you to relax muscles and the mind; to change your attitude towards back pain; and to help identify, cope with and resolve mental and physical stresses and emotional issues that may be causing the muscles to contract. *Before commencing any program, discuss it thoroughly with your physician and obtain his/her approval.*

Do not be discouraged by the time the programs take. Most of it is fun, necessary to the management and control of pain, and designed to improve the quality of life. Moreover, you can combine goal activities such as humor and walking, or music with other walks or relaxation techniques. This reduces the time commitment markedly.

If a particular goal and associated activity is required, the following abbreviation will be noted next to the goal: LF refers to long form, SF refers to short form, and DO refers to design-your-own. Where there is a difference in frequency between programs it will be discussed. Below is a chart that lists the elements of each program for comparison at a glance:

The Three Programs Compared

Each skill, goal, or activity will be listed in the Long Form column. R will appear in the Short Form or Design-Your-Own columns if an element is also required in that program. NR will mean not required. O will appear after a program component if it is optional. All elements listed in the LF column are required, unless an O appears.

Long Form	Short Form	Design-Your-Own
Positive thinking	R	R
Affirmations	R	R
Prayer(O)	O	O
Imagery	R	R
Self-Hypnosis	O	O
Journalizing	R	R
Humor	R	NR
Music	R	NR
Meditation	R	NR
Body sensing	R	R
Uncontracting Muscles	R	R
Deep breathing	R	NR
Somatics	R	R
Feldenkrais	R	R
Exercise	R	R
Walking	R	R
Acupressure	NR	NR
Proper Form	R	R
Self-massage (O)	O	O
Aromatherapy	R	O
Herbal bath (O)	O	O
Pain Flare-up techniques	R	R
Vocational goals	R	R

Long Form	Short Form	Design-Your-Own
Yoga	R	R
Vocational goals	R	R
Lunch/breaks with co-workers	R	NR
Outing with family	R	NR
Outing with friends	R	NR
Weekend bike ride (O)	O	O
Comedy walk	R	NR
Swim (O)	O	O
Hobby	R	NR
Old movies/books (O	O	O
Join the Internet (O)	O	O
Diet, weight control, nutrition	R	R
Vitamins and supplements	R	R
Medications	R	R
Doctor's visits	R	R
Professional appointments	R	R

Please read the following for specific details on how to carry out these goals, associated activities, and frequency with which they should be done. Refer back to appropriate chapters if necessary.

Attitude Goals

Positive Thinking: (LF-SF-DO) *A positive, I-can-do-it attitude is an absolute must.* To ensure a positive frame of mind, use any of the techniques specified in Chapter 4. If you get in trouble, (that is discouraged or frustrated) use the thought-stopping techniques noted in that chapter, or go back and read the section in Chapter 1, "Gathering the Harvest" to remind yourself what you gain in these programs in the long run, or read Chapter 1 on discipline and commitment again for some incentive and motivation.

Frequency: Daily, every waking minute of the day.

Affirmations: (LF-SF-DO) Daily affirmations are powerful attitude changers. Your pain experience will be changed for the good when you use them. Write at least 2 daily affirmations on cards, post them on a mirror and take them with you wherever you go.

Frequency: Daily, taking about 10 minutes. Take time to write the affirmations using the guidelines from Chapter 4 and then repeat or read the affirmations frequently throughout the day.

Prayer: (Optional) Use any of the techniques suggested in Chapter 13, or any prayers you are already using and/or familiar with.

Frequency: Daily, taking about 5 minutes a day. If you choose, attend one religious service per week. Praying upon waking and before going to sleep is effective.

PAIN MANAGEMENT GOALS

Mental Means of Pain Relief

Imagery and/or Self Hypnosis: (LF-SF-DO) Whenever you feel pain, use the imagery techniques suggested in Chapter 6.

Frequency: Daily application of imagery techniques when pain strikes. This will take about 20 minutes. For those in the long form program we suggest both imagery and self-hypnosis.

Journaling: (LF-SF-DO) Identifying mental and physical stressors and emotional issues, planning their resolution, and resolving them, if possible.

Frequency: Daily, make entries in the daily pain tracking journal; and at the end of the week, complete the summary. Don't forget to construct an action plan to resolve the stressors. For the long form program do the program suggested by the individual who cured himself of chronic back pain, specified in Chapter 3.

Humor Therapy: (LF-SF) Spend 15 minutes a day listening to something funny. In the evening read humor and pick out two jokes to tell throughout the next day.

Frequency: Daily, 15 minutes listening to, and 15 minutes reading humor, and picking two best jokes. For those on the long form program, $1/2$ hour to an hour of watching comedy on TV is recommended.

Music: (LF) Listening to favorite music as often and much as you can, combined with other goal activities, such as imagery or walking.

Frequency: Daily, 30 minutes a day, and as a background to other activities.

Meditation: (LF-SF) Spend at least 15 minutes daily meditating. You can also incorporate meditation with walking.

Frequency: Daily, 15 minutes.

Body Sensing: (LF-SF-DO) Sense what is happening in the body and keep your muscles in a state of relaxation as much as you can. Your back should be flat and loose with no muscles in spasm. Observe proper standing and sitting specified in Chapter 19.

Deep Breathing: (LF-SF) Practice deep breathing techniques whenever you feel anxious, or are in pain.

Frequency: Daily, as needed, for about 5 minutes at a time.

The Physical Means of Pain Relief

Exercise: (LF-SF-DO) Exercise is critical. Start with the beginning gentle workout for the first few weeks. Do the full workout every day; but do the aerobic and strengthening exercises every other day. We strongly suggest a few morning stretches in the shower after about 10 minutes of warm water.

Frequency: Daily in accord with this schedule:

Feldenkrais & Somatics Exercises: Somatics after a bath or shower in the morning; Feldenkrais later in the day. Somatics before bed.

Full Workout: Every other day.

Stretching & Back Exercises: Daily.

Yoga Workout: Every other day for LF and two days a week for SF

Walking: (LF-SF-DO) Walking is one of the most effective exercises for relieving back pain. Incorporate meditation, repeat affirmations or listening to humor while walking.

Frequency: LF—30 minutes in the morning, and 30 minute walk after lunch and dinner. SF& DO—One 30 minute walk during the day.

Acupressure Workouts: (LF) Acupressure workouts have a cumulative effect on mood and pain control. Make a tape of the most effective points with background music by narrating the location of points and type of pressure to use.

Frequency: Daily, using the acupressure mood uplifter and chronic pain workouts in Chapter 21.

Proper Form: (LF-SF-DO) Practice proper standing, sitting and walking postures at all times. Stretch frequently throughout the day using those that you find release muscle tension best. Rest your back using the exercises discussed in the Proper Form chapter.

Frequency: Constantly, throughout the day. Every 30 minutes, stand up and do your favorite stretches if you have been sitting.

Uncontract Muscles: (LF-SF-DO) Use Fold and Hold and other Touch for Health techniques discussed in Chapter 26 to uncontract muscles.

Frequency: Daily, as needed.

Self Massage: (Optional) Treat yourself to a self-massage as a means of relaxing all muscles.

Frequency: Every other day, when you are not doing your full workout.

Herbal Bath: (Optional) Treat yourself to a relaxing 15-20 minute herbal bath.

Frequency: On the day you do your full workout, take an herbal bath to relax your muscles.

Flare-Up Pain Control Goals: (LF-SF-DO)

This is the emergency plan for flare-ups. These are supplemental mental and physical means of pain relief to be used in addition to other pain management skills that are part of the program. Generally you will use your most effective technique first, followed immediately by other techniques until the pain abates. The order and length of time to apply the physical and/or mental means of pain control is up to you. Frequency, as needed, during a flare up, until the pain lessens and you calm down physically and emotionally. Choose the ones that are most effective for you, based on past experience as reflected in your charts. Make a copy of your flare-up plan and have it and the materials you need with you at all times.

Do not get discouraged. You have tools to deal with the pain. Move on, and above all, do not let the flare-up stop you from doing what you want to do and maintain a positive attitude.

Vocational Goals: LF-SF-DO

Work or Volunteer Work: If you have a job, work every day. Set sub-goals in work, including additional projects you can accomplish, while also raising performance levels. Work is an important pain relief method because it is a strong distraction. When you return to work make sure you have a flare-up plan and the equipment you need to effectuate it. As an alternative try and set up a business where you can work out of your house.

If you do not have a job, volunteer in the community. Your services will be needed. Try the local hospital, library, or anywhere else that wants help. As with work goals, set sub-goals in your volunteer activities, develop an action plan for them and make sure you accomplish these goals

On the weekends engage in self study or attend classes.

Frequency: Daily work or volunteering five days a week is a must. Ideally you should spend 8 hours a day at work, and 3 hours a day volunteering if you do not have a job, with the remaining 2 hours a day devoted to finding a job. If you are off work, but can return, return in accord with what your doctor advises.

Social Goals

Coming out of isolation and connecting with others is vitally important to the pain management program. The more you can do the better. Try these suggestions.

Lunch and Coffee Breaks With Your Co-Workers or Co-Volunteers: (LF-SF)
Frequency: 3 times a week, minimum, preferably 5 times a week.

Social Outing With Family: (LF-SF) Involving your family in your pain management program will give you great satisfaction and support. Suggested activities include a picnic, bike ride, or trip to the movies.
Frequency: Once a week at a minimum, preferably 2-3 times a week.

Social Outing With Friends or Another Couple: (LF-SF) Visiting with friends also reconnects you. Suggested activities include: shopping, movies, lunch or dinner, or events such as sports, games, or theater.
Frequency: Once a week for SF, twice a week for LF.

Recreational Goals

This is another fun part of the program. Five recreational goals should be chosen at a minimum, three of which must involve exercise for the long form program, two for the short form program and your choice for design-your-own programs. Here are some suggestions:

Weekend Bike Ride: (Optional) Bike rides are an excellent way to loosen muscles.
Frequency: $1/2$ hour bike ride each day of the weekend.

The Comedy Walk: (LF-SF) How about a daily comedy walk? If you have a treadmill, take a slow walk on it while watching a favorite sitcom. If you like the outdoors, audio tape your favorite sitcom and use a Walkman.
Frequency: $1/2$ hour daily.

The Twice Weekly Swim: (Optional) Swimming is one of the best exercises for chronic back pain. If you have access to a pool, do laps in accord with your doctor's recommendation.
Frequency: Twice weekly.

Develop A Hobby: (LF-SF) Finding a hobby you enjoy is a great distraction from pain. Whether it be model planes, sewing, listening to comedy, or whatever, find what pleases and distracts.

Frequency: 5 times a week, at least ¹/₂ hour a day, for long form program and 2 times a week for short form program.

Catching Up on Old Movies or Books: (Optional) clearly distracts you from pain. *Frequency:* 5 hours a week, over 5 days.

Computer Usage: (Optional) One of the most satisfying activities author Miller has done is to become proficient in computer usage, and surfing the Internet. This a great distraction where you learn a lot and meet great people. *Frequency:* 5 hours a week, spread over 5 days.

Diet, Weight Control, Vitamins, Herb & Nutrition: (LF-SF-DO) After discussing our recommendations in Chapter 27 with your physician (relative to diet, weight control, vitamins, herbs, supplements, and amino acids) develop a defined program to be adhered to daily.

Health Care Resources: (LF-SF-DO)

Medications: No doubt your physician has prescribed medicine to help manage pain. Medicine can play a very important role. *Frequency:* Take as prescribed.

Doctor's Visits: Once your condition has been diagnosed as chronic pain, you need not run to the doctor with every flare-up, unless the flare-up is serious. *Frequency:* Visit the doctor in accordance with scheduled appointments. Avoid emergency room or other doctor visits during flare ups, unless the flare-up is serious and of a different character than previous ones.

Other Professional Treatments, such as physical therapy or psychotherapy, may be part of your pain management program. Keep these appointments; they are designed to help you.

The Goal Setting and Accomplishment Pain Management Contracts

We have included a goal accomplishment chart for each of the recommended programs. This chart has the mandated elements of each program on it. We call it a pain management contract. Keep the chart with you and fill it out daily as you accomplish each of the goals and associated activities. Make copies of the chart and start tracking progress.

Setting and accomplishing goals is the key to reducing and potentially eliminating chronic back pain. Do it every day without fail and begin to reap its benefits in reduced pain. If these recommendations are not in accord with your condition, per your doctor's advice, pick alternate goal activities that your physician concurs with. We encourage you to try as many as the pain relief suggestions you want, provided you clear them with your doctor. *Be persistent and do not be discouraged.* Remember that taking control of your pain rather than letting it ruin or victimize you is the only way to go. Successful pain management takes work, patience, self-discipline and a positive attitude. Be a winner and remember that a quitter never wins and a winner never quits.

Finally, make sure you bring with you the necessary equipment wherever you are to accomplish your program and manage your pain. If you need to take a time out to do stretching or manage a flare-up, do so. Those around you will clearly understand and support your efforts.

Summing Up the Main Principles

1. Chronic back pain is a true disease that can be appropriately managed with an effective pain management program.

2. Chronic back pain is generally caused by involuntary, habituated muscle contractions induced by stress and emotional issues as well as ongoing reaction to the pain.

3. The object of the recommended programs is to restore you to a full functioning life doing those things that you want to do and accomplish.

4. The recommended programs should significantly reduce or eliminate your pain through 1. distraction; 2. methods to relieve your anxiety; 3. an understanding of the source of your pain; 4. exercise programs designed to uncontract, strengthen muscles and make them more flexible; and 5. highly effective mental and physical means to block the pain signal's transmission to the brain.

5. A positive belief that the methods in this book will assist in pain relief is essential to success.

6. Removing negative thoughts and negativism in your life and replacing it with a more optimistic attitude through positive thoughts are all important to pain relief.

7. Your declared intention to manage and relieve your pain will result in pain relief.

8. Recognizing and resolving your nonphysical and physical stressors will markedly assist in pain relief.

9. The management of pain through the participation in goal setting and accomplishment is highly effective in managing and potentially resolving

chronic pain issues.

10. You must take control of pain to manage and defeat it before it manages and defeats you.

11. A positive attitude together with self-responsibility, patience, commitment, and hard work in utilizing a pain management program will lead to positive results and a quality-of-life enhancing accomplishment, joy, and happiness.

12. Nothing can defeat the human spirit and will power.

13. Significant pain relief or a pain-free life, *can* be accomplished, provided it is *your* vision, *your* determination, and you are willing to do what it takes in terms of time and effort to accomplish it.

14. Knowledge is power. This book puts an enormous amount of knowledge at your fingertips to help you overcome your pain and suffering.

15. The choice is yours: *Be a victim of pain or manage it and return to a happy, full-functioning life.*

AFTERWORD

A journey of a thousand miles begins with the first step, and you have taken that first step towards pain relief by reading this book. To those of you in pain, this book should be heartening because it was written by someone like you—a back pain sufferer. To those of you in the healing professions, this book should also be encouraging because it was written by a back pain patient who worked in full partnership with his doctors and other health care professionals. This book represents hundreds of hours of footwork, reading, research, schooling in and experience with back pain relief. It's all here for you in one place. We sincerely hope that back pain patients and those helping pain patients to find relief will use this book as a guide along the road to full recovery. We wish you well in your journey.

SELF PAIN MANAGEMENT CONTRACT / LONG FORM

(Place a check mark in the appropriate box as goals are completed-can combine activities)

Week of: _____

Goal Activities	Frequency	Mon	Tues	Wed	Thur	Fri	Sat	Sun
1. **Attitude Goals**								
a. Positive Thinking	Daily							
b Affirmations	Daily							
2. **Vocational Goals**								
a Work or Volunteer Work	Monday thru Friday							
b.Classes or Self Study	Weekends							
3. **Social Goals**								
a Family Activities	Twice a Week							
b Activities with Friends	Twice a Week							
c.Coffee/Lunch-Co-workers	Three Times a Week							
4. **Recreational Goals**								
a. Walking	Three Times Daily							
b. Hobbies	Five Times a Week							
c .Yoga	Four Times a Week							
5. **Pain Management Skills**								
a Imagery & Self Hypnosis	Daily							
b Journaling	Daily							
c Humor & Music	Daily							
d.Exercise Program	Daily							
e Meditation	Daily							
f. Feldenkrais & Somatics	Daily							
g.Proper Form & Body Sensing	Daily							
h. Deep Breathing	Daily							
i. Uncontract Muscles	Daily							
j. Aromatherapy	Daily							
k. Acupressure	Daily							
6. **Pain Control Flare-Up Skills**	**Choose Techniques**							
a	Daily as Needed							
b	Daily as Needed							
c.	Daily as Needed							
7. **Diet, Vitamins, Herbs Nutrition Goals**								
a.Vitamins & Supplements	Daily							
b. Weight Loss	Daily							
c.Healthy Diet	Daily							
8. **Health Care Resources**								
a Keep Health Appointments	As Scheduled							
b No Emerency Room or Dr.	Daily							
c Take Medications	Daily							

Completed: _____ (Signature and Date)

SELF PAIN MANAGEMENT CONTRACT / SHORT FORM
(Place a check mark in the appropriate box as goals are completed-can combine activities)

Week of: _____

Goal Activities	Frequency	Mon	Tues	Wed	Thur	Fri	Sat	Sun
1. **Attitude Goals**								
a. Positive Thinking	Daily							
b Affirmations	Daily							
2. **Vocational Goals**								
a Work or Volunteer Work	Monday thru Friday							
3. **Social Goals**								
a Family Activities	Once a Week							
b Activities with Friends	Once a Week							
c.Coffee/Lunch-Co-workers	Twice a Week							
4. **Recreational Goals**								
a. Walking	One time daily							
b. Hobbies	Two Times a Week							
c .Yoga	Two Times a Week							
5. **Pain Management Skills**								
a Imagery or Self Hypnosis	Daily							
b Journaling	Daily							
c Humor & Music	Daily							
d.Exercise Program	Daily							
e Meditation	Daily							
f. Feldenkrais & Somatics	Daily							
g Proper Form & Body Sensing	Daily							
h. Deep Breathing	Daily							
i. Aromatherapy	Daily							
j. Uncontract Muscles	Daily							
6. **Pain Control Flare-Up Skills**	**Choose Techniques**							
	Daily as Needed							
	Daily as Needed							
	Daily as Needed							
7. **Diet, Vitamins, Herbs Nutrition Goals**								
a.Vitamins & Supplements	Daily							
b Weight Loss	Daily							
c.Healthy Diet	Daily							
8. **Health Care Resources**								
a Keep Health Appointments	As Scheduled							
b No Emerency Room or Dr.	Daily							
c Take Medications	Daily							

Completed: _____ (Signature and Date)

SELF PAIN MANAGEMENT CONTRACT / DESIGN YOUR OWN
(Place a check mark in the appropriate box as goals are completed-can combine activities)
Week of: _____

Goal Activities	Frequency	Mon	Tues	Wed	Thur	Fri	Sat	Sun
1. **Attitude Goals**								
a. Positive Thinking	Daily							
b Affirmations	Daily							
2. **Vocational Goals**								
a Work or Volunteer Work	Monday thru Friday							
3. **Social Goals**								
a. Breaks/Lunch-Co-workers								
4. **Recreational Goals**								
a. Walking	One time daily							
5. **Pain Management Skills**								
a Imagery or Self Hypnosis	Daily							
b Journaling	Daily							
c.Proper Form & Body Sensing	Daily							
d.Exercise Program	Daily							
e.Deep Breathing	Daily							
f.Feldenkrais & Somatics	Daily							
g.Uncontract Muscles	Daily							
6. **Pain Control Flare-Up Skills**	**Choose Techniques**							
7. **Diet, Vitamins, Herbs Nutrition Goals**								
a.Vitamins & Supplements	Daily							
b.Weight Loss	Daily							
c.Healthy Diet	Daily							
8. **Health Care Resources**								
a Keep Health Appointments	As Scheduled							
b No Emercency Room or Dr.	Daily							
c Take Medications	Daily							

Completed: _____ (Signature and Date)

APPENDIX A

OBTAINING UPDATES ON THE INTERNET
& CONTACTING THE AUTHORS

WITH THE PUBLICATION OF THIS BOOK the authors are establishing a home page in the World Wide Web section of the Internet. The home page will contain a wealth of information: book updates, additional pain relieving techniques and products, the latest in back pain research and developments, a bibliography of relevant books and tapes, the results of an Internet survey on techniques from around the world, and links to other web pages that relate to chronic pain, including back pain.

The web address is: www.backpainalternatives.com.

E-mail the authors at RMiller141@aol.com, or by writing to us at:

Back Pain Relief Alternatives
969 G Edgewater Blvd. #358
Foster City, California 94404

We look forward to hearing from you with your success stories as well as any back pain relief techniques that you have found to work. With your permission, we would like to share them with others in pain around the world.

APPENDIX B

USING A COMPUTER AND LIBRARY TO OBTAIN FURTHER INFORMATION ON TECHNIQUES TO RELIEVE BACK PAIN

THIS BOOK CONTAINS the authors' views on the most effective modalities for back pain relief. However, there are other alternative therapies that have proved useful in reducing or relieving back pain. These include: (1) acupuncture; (2) biofeedback training; (3) chiropractic; (4) craniosacral therapy; (5) homeopathy; (6) osteopathy; and (7) rolfing. These therapies require the services of a qualified practitioner. To learn more, read about them in the library or check them out on-line.

A home computer with a modem opens a whole world of on-line resources. The Internet contains an enormous amount of useful information on back pain relief. Follow these simple steps to get onto the information super highway:

1. Log onto the Internet.

2. Go to the World Wide Web and type in www.search.com.

3. This site has some of the best search engines on the Web. By typing in a word or series of words on these search engines you will discover numerous sites. Try these words or phrases: pain, back pain, chronic pain, back pain relief, holistic medicine, alternative medicine, and holistic health. Many of the sites have links to other sites. Click on the sites that look most interesting to you.

4. View and print important information on selected pages.

Additionally, you can read and post messages in the Usenet section of the Internet in news groups such as misc.health, alternative and alt.support, chronic-pain.

America On Line, in its Health Forum, contains a comprehensive section on pain relief. In addition to articles on back pain, chronic pain and holistic alternatives to dealing with pain, there are excellent discussion groups on these issues. Through the posting of messages relating to back pain you will be able to dialogue with others who have chronic back pain. No doubt they will provide further suggestions to assist you in managing pain. Check out their software library also to discover a number of special programs and books covering natural alternatives for pain relief.

APPENDIX C

PERMISSIONS

We gratefully acknowledge the following authors and publishers for allowing us to reprint from, quote or discuss concepts from their books:

The Book of Pain Relief, Leon Chaitow, published by Thorsons, an imprint of HarperCollins Publishers, Ltd., London.

The Healing Power of Humor, Allen Klein, reprinted by permission of Putnam/Jeremy P. Tarcher, Inc., copyright (c) 1989 by Allen Klein.

Mastering Pain, Dr. Richard Sternbach, reprinted by permission of the Putnam Publishing Group, copyright (c) 1987 by Dr. Richard Sternbach.

Life Without Pain, Dr. R. M. Linchitz, (extracted from pages 91-96) (c) 1987 Richard M. Linchitz M.D., reprinted by permission of Addison-Wesley Longman Publishing Company, Inc.

The Reflexology Workbout, Stephanie Rick, copyright (c) 1986 by Rita Aero and Stephanie Rick, reprinted by permission of Harmony Books, a division of Crown Publishers, Inc.

Anatomy of an Illness as Perceived by a Patient: Reflections on Healing and Regeneration, Norman Cousins, copyright (c) 1979 by W. W. Norton & Company, Inc, reprinted by permission of W. W. Norton & Company, Inc.

Healing Words, Larry Dossey, M. D. Copyright (c) 1993, HarperCollins.

Prescription for Nutritional Healing, James and Phyllis Balch, Avery Publishing Group.

The Portable Life 101, Peter McWilliams, Prelude Press.

Choose to Live Your Life Fully, Susan Smith Jones, Celestial Arts Publishing.

Stretching, Bob Anderson, Shelter Publications.

Tai Chi-Ten Minutes to Health, Chia Siew Pang and Goh Ewe Hock, CRCS Publications.

Relaxation Techniques, Jenny Sutcliffe, People's Medical Society.

Journey of Awakening, Ram Dass, Bantam/Doubleday Dell

Healing Music, Watson and Drury, Prism Press

Quantum Healing, Deepak Chopra, Bantam/Doubleday Dell

The Back Pain Book: A Self-Help Guide for the Daily Relief of Back and Neck Pain, Mike Hage, Peachtree Publishers.

Your Body Believes Every Word You Say, Barbara Hoberman Levine, Aslan Publishing.

Hot Water Therapy, Horay and Harp, New Harbinger Publications.

Walking Through Stress-Meditation in Motion, Dick Harding, Cassandra Press.

The Chronic Pain Control Workbook, llen Mohr Catalano, New Harbinger Press.

The Relaxation and Stress Reduction Workbook, Martha Davis, Elizabeth Eshelman, & Matthew McKay, New Harbinger Press.

Hands on Healing, the Editors of Prevention Magazine, Rodale Press.

90 Seconds to Pain Relief: The Fold and Hold Method, Dr. Dale Anderson, Chronimed Publishers.

Life Without Pain, Komar and Brad Steiger, Berkeley Publishing Corp.

Touch for Health, John F. Thie, D.C.

Become Pain Free with Touch for Health, John McGuire.

APPENDIX D

ABOUT THE AUTHORS

Robert H. Miller

Mr. Miller, an attorney and member of the senior executive service, is employed by the National Labor Relations Board as Regional Director of Region 20 in San Francisco. He received a B.S. from Pennsylvania State University and his law degree from Dickinson School of Law. Additionally, he did graduate work in labor law at Georgetown University. Recently, he became a California Certified Holistic Health Counselor and is currently studying to be a Kinesiology/Touch For Health practitioner. He also authored *Bicycle Trails of Southern California.* Miller resides in the San Francisco Bay Area with his wife, Bonnie, and his son, Jason.

Christine A. Opie

Ms. Opie is a writing teacher at California State University, Hayward, where she coaches developing writers. She received her B.A. in History from Sacramento State University and her M.A. in English from San Francisco State University. In addition to her training as an English teacher, Ms. Opie also received her Master Hypnotist certificate. She has taught self-hypnosis for stress reduction, and has made hypnosis tapes for family, friends, and co-workers. Ms. Opie brings to this book twenty years of teaching experience in Africa, Asia and the U.S. She has co-authored a textbook entitled, *Writing Proficiency Workbook.* She resides in the San Francisco Bay Area with her cat, Kiki.

Dr. William Brose

Dr. Brose, a recognized authority in pain management, is the Founder and former Director of the Stanford University Medical Center Pain Management Service. Currently he is an Associate Professor of Anesthesiology at Stanford University Medical Center, and is in private practice at Alpha-Omega Pain Medicine Associates in Palo Alto, California.

APPENDIX E

CONTENTS OF CDs AND HOW TO ORDER THEM

Use the order form at the back of the book to order the CDs. The cost is $14.95 plus $1.75 for shipping and handling. California residents include $1.23 for sales tax. Payment can be made by personal check, money order or Visa and Master Card. Allow 4 weeks for delivery. Send completed order form to:

BACK PAIN RELIEF ALTERNATIVES
969 G. Edgewater Blvd. #358, Foster City, CA 94404

CONTENTS:
CD #1— *The Mental Means of Pain Relief*

Title	Track #
Introduction	1
Eye fixation	2
Waves of Relaxation	3
Complete Induction (hypnosis)	4
Lemon Visualization	5
Body Visualization	6
Image of Your Pain (visualization)	7
Pain Relief Imagery	8
Breath Awareness Practice	9
Breathing with Affirmations	10
Meditation	11
Laughter	12

CD #2 —*The Physical Means of Pain Relief*

Title	Track #
Introduction	1
Warm Up	2
Special Strengthening	3
Introduction to Weights	4

ORDER FORM FOR AUDIO CDs

COST OF 2 AUDIO CDs $14.95
SALES TAX (8.25%) $ 1.23   (Calif. residents only)
SHIPPING & HANDLING $ 1.75

TOTAL   **$16.70 or ($17.93 for California)**

(PLEASE ALLOW 2-4 WEEKS FOR DELIVERY)

METHOD OF PAYMENT: (PLEASE CHECK ONE)

CHECK( ) (Make checks payable to: Back Pain Relief Alternatives, LLC)
MONEY ORDER( )   VISA( )   MASTERCARD( )

NAME ON CARD: _____

ACCOUNT NUMBER: _____

EXPIRATION DATE :_____

SIGNATURE _____

SEND ORDER FORM TO:
BACK PAIN RELIEF ALTERNATIVES, LLC.
969 G EDGEWATER BLVD. #358
FOSTER CITY, CA 94404

SHIP TO: Please Print

NAME:_____

ADDRESS:_____APT# _____

CITY, STATE, ZIP:_____